Health Promotion

Edited by Mukadder Mollaoğlu

Published in London, United Kingdom

Health Promotion
http://dx.doi.org/10.5772/intechopen.98025
Edited by Mukadder Mollaoğlu

Contributors
Eva-Carin Lindgren, Linn Håman, Katarina Haraldsson, Alf Trojan, Marwa Khalfalli, Jerome Verny, Aishat Alaran, Fahd Khalid-Salako, Yusff Adebisi, Abubakar Badmos, Oluwaseyifunmi Oladipo, Zainab Onibon, Don Eliseo Prisno Iii, Vanessa Ferreira, Ivy Scorzi Cazelli Pires, Milton Cosme Ribeiro, Vivian Vimarlund, Diana Zandi, Peter Delobelle, Joyce Mashamba, Suraya Mohamed, Hans Onya, Annikki Arola, Dabota Yvonne Buowari, Amornrat Ratanasiri, Thawalsak Ratanasiri, Somnuk Apiwantanagul, Bangonsri Jindawong, Thanawan Sirisuk, Chanchanok Aramrat, Papia Sultana, Mukadder Mollaoğlu, Songül Mollaoglu, Safiye Yanmış

First published in London, United Kingdom, 2022 by IntechOpen
IntechOpen is the global imprint of INTECHOPEN LIMITED, registered in England and Wales, registration number: 11086078, 5 Princes Gate Court, London, SW7 2QJ, United Kingdom

British Library Cataloguing-in-Publication Data
A catalogue record for this book is available from the British Library

Additional hard and PDF copies can be obtained from orders@intechopen.com

Health Promotion
Edited by Mukadder Mollaoğlu
p. cm.
Print ISBN 978-1-80355-546-1
Online ISBN 978-1-80355-547-8
eBook (PDF) ISBN 978-1-80355-548-5

Meet the editor

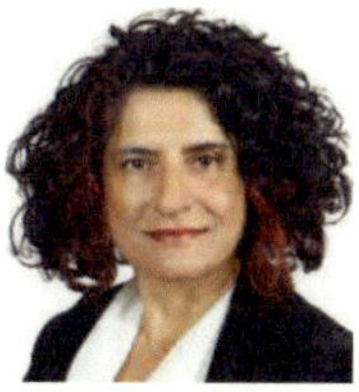

Professor Dr. Mukadder Mollaoğlu is a member of the Faculty of Health Sciences, Sivas Cumhuriyet University, Turkey. Her research interests are health promotion, care management in chronic diseases, quality of life, life satisfaction, home care, needs of caregivers, improving self-care activities in chronic diseases, self-efficacy, medicine, and nursing ethics. Her research studies have been published in many high-impact journals and have received numerous citations. She has also published several books and book chapters. Professor Mollaoğlu received two first prizes for her work on life satisfaction and home care in chronic diseases, one in Sweden (Malmö) and the other in France (Strasbourg). In addition, she received the Lütfi Abay Culture and Education Foundation (LAKEV) science award in 2020 for research in the field of health sciences.

Contents

Preface

Health promotion has started to attract increasing attention not only from health professionals but also from the public. Indeed, the need for health promotion programs concerns all of us. Health promotion is the process of enabling people to increase control over and improve their health. This process improves the well-being of the individual. *Health Promotion* covers actions and practices aimed at creating behavioral change for the protection and improvement of health. These consist of health education as well as organizational, economic, and environmental support.

Ensuring that healthy lifestyle behaviors spread to individuals, families, groups, and societies is one of the important goals of improving health. With this understanding, attempts are being made to improve the personal choices and social responsibilities of individuals. Thus, people will be able to participate in practices that will enable them to improve their own health. In addition, people will take responsibility for their actions to maintain their own health.

Health promotion ensures the protection and development of health and psychological, social, and physical wellbeing, which is achieved through the collective efforts of individuals, society, public institutions and organizations, and non-governmental organizations. For this reason, attention is drawn to the importance of the determinants of health by pointing out that it is not enough to focus only on changing the behavior of the individual in health promotion actions in this book. In these actions, the importance of planning, implementing, and evaluating health education and health promotion programs with systematic approaches and the implementation of public health policies are emphasized.

In the 21st century, health-related changes such as climate change, globalization, digitalization, and the emergence of new contagious and non-communicable diseases continue as important problems that threaten the health of societies. The examples of health promotion in the book show how people are affected by the cultural, social, and environmental factors in which they live. At the same time, it shows that the values, beliefs, attitudes, and behaviors of target groups have an impact on health promotion. The book also highlights the need to create programs based on theories, models, and approaches that provide information and guide the design, implementation, and evaluation process of health promotion programs for health promotion professionals. I hope this book will contribute to achieving these goals and provide guidance and inspiration for a healthier world.

I would like to thank all the authors who contributed to this book and the staff at IntechOpen who provided invaluable cooperation and support throughout the publication process.

Dr. Mukadder Mollaoğlu,
Professor,
Health Sciences Faculty,
Sivas Cumhuriyet University,
Sivas, Turkey

Section 1

Health Promotion in Current Perspective

Chapter 1

Health Promotion: Trajectory and Current Perspectives

Vanessa Alves Ferreira, Ivy Scorzi Cazelli Pires and Milton Cosme Ribeiro

Abstract

Health promotion is linked to the living conditions of populations. In the last 40 years, health promotion reappears as a promising strategy for the field of Public Health. The health promotion movement emerged more vigorously from the 1970s onwards in developed countries—Canada, the United States and Western Europe. It is particularly in Canada that the concept of health promotion was revived, with the publication in 1974 of the Lalonde Report (A New Perspective on the Health of Canadians). This document placed health promotion at the level of strategic planning. The Lalonde Report has had a significant impact, providing insights into the recent health promotion movement across the world. Later, in 1978, the World Health Organization (WHO) held the 1st International Conference on Primary Health Care in Alma-Ata. This conference emphatically reaffirmed a broad concept of health. Health as a state of complete physical, mental and social well-being, not merely the absence of disease. This reconceptualization of health was fundamental in this process, as it served as the basis for the current health promotion movement. In this chapter, we intend to recover the trajectory and developments of the concept of health promotion and point out its future perspectives.

Keywords: health promotion, quality of life, sustainable development goals (ODS), COVID-19

1. Introduction

The first authors who made reference to the concept of health promotion were Winslow and Sigerist. Both related the term health promotion to the living conditions of populations. Leavell & Clark appropriated the concept when formulating the model of the natural history of the disease. According to the authors, preventive medicine would comprise three levels of prevention and health promotion would be included in the primary level, related to the health and well-being of individuals. In fact, the discourse of social medicine in the ninteenth century also maintained an approximation with health promotion, by correlating health and living conditions, through the works of authors such as Villermé, in France and Chadwick, in England. In this sense, the term health promotion is not recent [1].

The health promotion movement emerged more vigorously from the 1970s onwards in developed countries: Canada, the United States and Western Europe. It is particularly in Canada that the resumption of the concept of health promotion can be observed, with the publication in 1974 of the Lalonde Report—A New Perspective on the Health of Canadians [2]. This document placed health promotion at the level of strategic planning. This proposal aimed, above all, to face the high costs of medical care in the country. The Lalonde Report had a significant impact, enabling the unfolding of the modern health promotion movement around the world. Later, in 1978, the World Health Organization (WHO) held the First International Conference on Primary Health Care in Alma-Ata. This event had a significant impact on health systems around the world, establishing the goal of Health for All in the Year 2000. This conference emphatically reaffirmed a broad concept of health. Health as a state of complete physical, mental and social well-being and not merely the absence of disease. This reconceptualization of health was fundamental in this process because it served as the foundation for the current health promotion movement [3, 4].

Subsequently, the Canadian Ministry of Health and the WHO began to structure concepts and practices on health promotion, favoring the holding of the First International Conference on Health Promotion held in Ottawa, Canada, in 1986. This meeting resulted in the Charter of Ottawa, considered a benchmark for health promotion [2]. The conference brought together participants from all over the world and aimed to share experiences in the sector.

The Ottawa Charter defined five priority areas for action in health promotion: (1) healthy public policies; (2) creating healthy environments; (3) reinforcement of community action; (4) development of personal skills and (5) reorientation of health services. Also in this Charter, the prerequisites for health are described: peace, education, housing, food, income, healthy ecosystem, social justice and equity. Health promotion therefore incorporates an expanded notion of health and comes closer to the idea of quality of life. In this approach, health would be the result of a broad spectrum associated with quality of life, comprising a set of values, such as: social justice, education, income, housing, food, nutrition, work, among others [5, 6].

Quality of life, in turn, would be a notion related to the degree of satisfaction of individuals with their family, social and environmental environment. For Minayo et al. ([7], p. 8) "the term encompasses many meanings, which reflect knowledge, experiences and values of individuals and collectivities that report to it in different times, spaces and histories, being, therefore, a social construction with the mark of cultural relativity ".

Other international conferences were held and provided further discussion on the topic of health promotion, as presented below:

- II International Conference on Health Promotion was held in Adelaide, Australia in 1988, whose central theme was healthy public policies. This meeting discussed the impact of public policies on the health of populations. The conference identified four priority areas to promote immediate action on healthy public policies: support for women's health; food and nutrition; tobacco and alcohol and the creation of health-friendly environments.

- III International Conference on Health Promotion was held in the city of Sundsval, Sweden in 1991, where the theme of favorable environments for health or healthy environments was discussed, not restricted to the physical or natural dimension, but the political, social, economic and social dimensions. More favorable to the health of populations.

- IV International Conference on Health Promotion took place in Jakarta, Indonesia in 1997. The theme defined for the meeting was "health promotion in the 21st century". The role of health determinants in identifying the directions and strategies needed to face the dilemmas and challenges of the twenty-first century was discussed.

- V International Conference on Health Promotion, held in Mexico in 2000, chose the theme "health promotion: towards greater equity" in which the responsibility of governments in proposing health policies was recognized. It was also highlighted the persistence of problems that demanded an urgent solution and, therefore, actions aimed at health, especially public health, were established.

- VI International Conference on Health Promotion held in Bankok, Thailand in 2005. The topic discussed was "health promotion in a globalized world" which sought to identify actions and commitments to address the determinants of health. The establishment of partnerships to promote social improvement was defended as a requirement of global development. In addition, the values and strategies of the Ottawa Charter were reaffirmed.

- VII International Conference on Health Promotion held in Nairobi, Kenya, in 2009, the impasses for implementation were discussed, inserting an effective mechanism for income distribution into the political and development agendas.

- VIII International Conference on Health Promotion held in Helsinki, Finland, in 2013. The Meeting was based on the Alma Ata Declaration on Primary Health Care (1978) and the Ottawa Charter for Health Promotion (1986). These documents identified intersectoral action and healthy public policies as central elements for health promotion and for achieving equity in health.

- IX International Conference on Health Promotion was held in 2016 in Shanghai, China. And its focus was to promote health through the adoption of measures consistent with achieving the Sustainable Development Goals (SDGs). The Declaration of the event contains four major themes and a series of commitments: (1) the adoption of political decisions in favor of the rights of women, displaced populations and the growing number of people affected by humanitarian and environmental crises. (2) Using governance strategies to promote well-being. (3) Recognition of cities and communities as essential environments for health. (4) Recognition of knowledge in health as a fundamental element for the promotion of equity in health. The Declaration ends with a "call to action" for the commitments made to accelerate the implementation of the SDGs through political commitment and financial investment in health promotion.

It is important that some conferences take place in different periods of time, but stand out as important events in the field of health promotion, among them: the Declaration of Santa Fé de Bogotá (1992); I Caribbean Health Promotion Conference, in the Caribbean (1993); Population Health Promotion in Canada (1996); Network of Mega Countries for Health Promotion (1998); V Latin American Conference on

Health Promotion and Health Education (2021). In addition to these, the United Nations Millennium Declaration held in New York in 2000 was equally important, where leaders set a goal to tackle and eliminate poverty in the world [4, 8]. **Table 1** below summarizes these events.

From the holding of international and regional conferences, it is observed that health promotion places the issue of health on the global public agenda as a priority for leaders at all levels and sectors, drawing attention to the consequences that the decisions taken by these countries have on global health. Thus, health promotion points to the need to build healthy public policies around the world; of creating favorable environments for people's health, alongside the development of personal skills and the reinforcement of community action [10]. It is important to emphasize that strategies and programs in the area of health promotion must adapt to the local needs and possibilities of each country and region, as well as taking into account the differences in their socio-cultural and economic systems.

Particularly, in the context of the organization of health policies, health promotion is understood as a powerful device for reformulating public policies that aim at the quality of life of populations. Health promotion would be a field of articulation with several areas that aim at people's quality of life within two approaches. The first

1974: A New Perspective on the Health of Canadians.
1977: Health for all in the year 2000—30th World Health Assembly.
1978: International Conference on Primary Health Care—Declaration of Alma Ata.
1986: I International Conference on Health Promotion (Canada)
1988: II World Conference on Health Promotion (Australia)
1991: III World Conference on Health Promotion (Sweden)
1992: I International Conference on Health Promotion in the Region of the Americas—Declaration of Bogotá (Colombia)
1993: I Conference on Health Promotion in the Caribbean (Caribbean)
1996: Population Health Promotion in Canada (1996)
1997: IV World Conference on Health Promotion (Indonesia)
1998: Network of Mega Countries for Health Promotion (Switzerland)
2000: V World Conference on Health Promotion (Mexico)
2000: United Nations Conference on the Millennium Development Goals (SDGs).
2002: III Latin American Conference on Health Promotion and Health Education (São Paulo, Brazil)
2005: VI World Conference on Health Promotion (Bangkok)
2008: Report of the Global Commission on Social Determinants of Health (WHO)
2009: VII World Conference on Health Promotion (Nairobi)
2012: United Nations Conference on Sustainable Development (Rio de Janeiro, Brazil)
2013: VIII World Conference on Health Promotion (Helsinki)
2015: United Nations Conference on Sustainable Development Goals (SDGs) and launch of Agenda 2030.
2016: IX World Conference on Health Promotion (Shanghai)
Source: adapted from Buss et al. [9].

Table 1.
Chronology of events in health promotion.

emphasizes the autonomy and accountability of individuals using health education as a strategy with a view to behavioral change. And the second, whose focus is broader and more comprehensive, seeking to identify and address the macro-determinants of the health-disease process through intersectoral actions. Health promotion therefore seeks to change the living conditions of people and populations so that they are dignified and adequate [6, 11].

For public policies to have coherence and practical effectiveness aimed at health promotion, they must be articulated to the different segments of society, involving civil society, the public and private sectors. The participation of society in this process implies the fight for health with the reduction of existing inequities in the access to infrastructure goods and services. For this, it is necessary to exercise empowerment, understood as an important strategy for strengthening and empowering people to claim their social rights [12].

In this direction, in order to achieve the objectives proposed by the health promotion strategy, coordinated action is necessary in the different sectors and among the multiple social actors: government, the health sector and other social and economic sectors, voluntary and non-governmental organizations, local authorities, industry and the media. Thus, people in all walks of life must be involved in this process as individuals, families and communities. Mediation between the population and the government, as well as training for the exercise of citizenship and social control are invaluable contributions to health promotion [5, 9].

We believe that it is through responsible public policies and initiatives to tackle the social determinants of health that health promotion takes place. Undoubtedly, its theoretical foundations and practices are directly related to governance, social responsibility and the fulfillment of global commitments assumed such as the 2030 Agenda and the Sustainable Development Goals—SDGs [9, 13], including the new challenges posed by the current COVID-19 pandemic.

2. Health promotion in the COVID-19 scenario

The COVID-19 pandemic, the biggest global health problem of this century, challenges scientific and political authorities to identify the most appropriate approaches from a clinical, epidemiological, political and socioeconomic point of view for its control and prevention. The main strategies adopted to face the COVID-19 pandemic involve: structuring and expanding hospital care in health systems, the use of telemedicine and the restriction of social contact.

Faced with the high pathogenicity and virulence of SARS-CoV-2, the governments of several countries seek to expand clinical beds and intensive care units dedicated to the treatment of severe cases of COVID-19 [14]. The use of telemedicine, in turn, aims to improve the response of health systems to the ongoing crisis. Its results show a greater capillarity and expansion of monitoring and health care, thus helping to monitor, detect and prevent, and to mitigate the impacts on health care indirectly related to COVID-19. In this way, such initiatives can reconfigure the future space of telemedicine in the practice of health services [15]. That is, when the pandemic is over, telemonitoring can continue to be used to provide more convenient and cost-effective care to patients. And yet, better prepare health systems for other pandemics that may arise in the future [16].

As for measures to restrict social contact, the most recommended are social distancing for the general population, isolation of confirmed and suspected cases, and the need to quarantine the contacts of those affected. Such restriction measures depend on the awareness and involvement of the population, as happened with countless other diseases of community control [14].

In this direction, experiences of articulation between scientific projects and the community to prevent the transmission of COVID-19 in the most vulnerable communities and the promotion of quality of life have been positive at this current moment. Such projects seek to build new health promotion practices and forms of knowledge production among the various social actors involved—epidemiologists, social scientists, infectologists, health professionals, patients and members of community groups, developing health actions of collective interest, enabling active participation of society in controlling this pandemic and other health problems. The actions involve health education, visits to scientific spaces, courses and workshops aimed at bringing science and society together in teaching, research and care spaces. These new forms of intervention in the COVID-19 epidemic may expand the scope of future public health actions because they broaden the look at the recent processes of social determination of health and the production of knowledge [17, 18].

Within this context, it is worth reflecting on the relevance not only of experiences of this nature, but on the other damage caused by COVID-19. Unemployment, hunger, social and psychological problems, violence and an increase in other diseases have been observed during the course of the pandemic [14].

According to PAHO [19], the pandemic intensified the weaknesses related to the guarantee of social rights in Latin American countries, impacting on the increase in unemployment rates, the reduction of income and the increase in situations of hunger and poverty. Also according to data from the Economic Commission for Latin America and the Caribbean—CEPAL [20], even before the Covid-19 pandemic, socially vulnerable groups such as rural women and the black population made up the indicators of poverty and extreme poverty in the American continent. The indigenous population was also affected by this situation, with a poverty rate of 46.7% in 2019 and extreme poverty at 17.3%. This poverty scenario intensified with the pandemic, and in 2020, the projection for the extreme poverty rate was 12.5% and 33.7% for the poverty rate, representing 209 million poor people by the end of that year in these countries. Countries. Such numbers have a direct influence on the increase in hunger of this population, as they impact on the purchasing power of food and all basic and essential human needs (CEPAL, 2020).

The complex social, ethical and political dimensions of the COVID-19 pandemic today serve as future lessons for building a more critical, ecological and democratic global health [21]. The reduction of social, health and environmental inequalities and injustices and the promotion of health and well-being are irremediable goals. And, therefore, they are characterized as enormous challenges for health systems around the world today.

3. Conclusion

Finally, to reach a potential for health and quality of life in contemporary times, it is necessary to increase investments in strategic health promotion actions. Thus, in the current context of the COVID-19 pandemic, investments in health have been mostly directed towards preventive and intervention measures. The priority has been to follow the recommendations of health organizations regarding the prevention of transmission of the new coronavirus: respiratory etiquette, social distancing, hand

and space hygiene [22]. In addition, they involve risk prevention actions for chronic diseases that, as the literature reveals, increase the severity and lethality of COVID-19 [23]. However, health promotion strategies are fundamental and should be encouraged at this time, due to the complex nature of the disease and the extension of the pandemic. Such strategies impose the establishment of a network of co-responsibilities in favor of life. And, they involve actions of reorganization and expansion of health services; Health education; encouraging healthy lifestyles and safe behaviors and creating healthy environments. In this direction, actions such as the one proposed by the World Health Organization [24]—"Food and nutrition tips during self-quarantine" to promote healthy eating during social isolation, is an example of the importance of health promotion actions in the current context. They reveal the new contours of the health promotion strategy during the COVID-19 health crisis around the world.

Health, as a social production of multiple and complex determination, requires public policies anchored in the perspective of health promotion. It fundamentally involves the establishment of a network of commitments and co-responsibilities in favor of life and the creation of the strategies necessary for it to be dignified and with quality [25]. Currently, due to the COVID-19 pandemic, investments have been increasing in curative and individual medical care, although it is identified that preventive measures, health promotion and improvement of living conditions are also being implemented, pointing out the new contours of actions of health promotion [9].

Author details

Vanessa Alves Ferreira[1,2]*, Ivy Scorzi Cazelli Pires[3,4] and Milton Cosme Ribeiro[5]

1 Sciences from the Oswaldo Cruz Foundation, FIOCRUZ/RJ, Brazil

2 Department of Nutrition, Federal University of Minas Gerais/UFMG, MG, Brazil

3 Food Science and Technology, Federal University of Viçosa/UFV, MG, Brazil

4 Nutrition Department, Federal University of Vales do Jequitinhonha e Mucuri, Brazil

5 Food Science from the Federal University of Minas Gerais/UFMG, Brazil

*Address all correspondence to: vanessa.nutr@gmail.com

References

[1] Ferreira VA, Magalhães R. Nutrition and health promotion: Current perspectives. Cadernos de Saúde Pública. 2007;**23**(7):1674-1681

[2] Brazil. Ministry of Health. Health Policy Secretariat. Health Promotion Project. Health Promotion Letters/ Ministry of Health, Health Policy Secretariat, Health Promotion Project. Brasília: Ministry of Health; 2002

[3] Czeresnia D, Freitas CM, organizers. Health Promotion: Concepts, Reflections, Trends. Rio de Janeiro: Editora Fiocruz; 2003

[4] World Health Organization (WHO). WHO Global Health Promotion Conferences. Washington: World Health Organization; 2022, 2020

[5] Buss PM. Health promotion and quality of life. Public Health Science. 2000;**5**:163-177

[6] Buss PM. An introduction to the concept of health promotion. In: Czeresnia D, Freitas CM, editors. Health Promotion: Concepts, Reflections, Trends. Rio de Janeiro: Editora Fiocruz; 2003. pp. 15-38

[7] Minayo MCM, Hartz ZMA, Buss PM. Quality of life and health: A necessary debate. Public Health Science. 2000;**5**:7-18

[8] Pereira de Paula DM, Aparecido de Faria M, Lacerda de Almeida JD. Multilateral cooperation in health: the Eighth International Conference on Health Promotion. Ibero-American Health Law Notebooks, [S. l.], v. 2, no. 2, p. 860-869, 2013. DOI: 10.17566/ciads.v2i2.127. Available at: https://www.cadernos.prodisa.fiocruz.br/index.php/cadernos/article/view/127 [Accessed: March 23, 2022]

[9] Buss P, de Hartz ZM, Pinto LF, Rocha CMF. Health promotion and quality of life: A historical perspective over the last 40 years (1980-2020). Science and Public Health. 2020;**25**(12):4723-4735

[10] CONASS (NATIONAL COUNCIL OF HEALTH SECRETARIES). Health Promotion: proposals from the National Council of Health Secretaries (CONASS) for its implementation as a public policy in Brazil. Brasilia. 2016. Available from: https://www.conass.org.br/promocao-da-saude

[11] Sonaglio RG, Lumertz J, Melo RC, Rocha CMF. Health promotion: Integrative review of concepts and experiences in Brazil. Journal of Nursing Health. 2019;**9**(3):e199301

[12] Heidmann ITSB, Almeida MCP, Boehs AE, Wosny AM, Monticelli M. Health promotion: Historical trajectory of its conceptions. Florianópolis. 2006;**15**(2):352-358

[13] World Health Organization (WHO). World Health Statistics 2019: Monitoring Health for the Sustainable Development Goals. Geneva: WHO; 2019

[14] Junior JPB, Morales MB. Community participation in the fight against COVID-19: Between utilitarianism and social justice. Canadian Public Health. 2020;**36**(8):e00151620

[15] Caetano R, Silva AB, Guedes ACM, Paiva CCN, Ribeiro GR, Santos DL, et al. Challenges and opportunities for teles health in times of the COVID-19 pandemic: A reflection on

spaces and initiatives in the Brazilian context. Canadian Public Health. 2020;**36**(5):e00088920

[16] Portnoy J, Waller M, Elliott T. Telemedicine in the Era of COVID-19. Journal of Allergy and Clinical Immunology Practice. 2020;**8**(5):1489-1491

[17] Kabad JF, Noal DS, Passos MFD, Melo BD, Pereira DR, Serpeloni F, et al. The experience of voluntary and collaborative work in mental health and psychosocial care in COVID-19. Canadian Public Health. 2020;**36**(9):e00132120

[18] de Souza CTV, de Santana CS, Ferreira P, Nunes JÁ, de Teixeira M, Gouvêa MIF. Cuidar in times of COVID-19: Lessons learned between science and society. Canadian Public Health. 2020;**36**(6):e00115020

[19] PAHO. Overview of Food and Nutrition Security in Latin America and the Caribbean. Santiago: Pan American Health Organization, Washington; 2020

[20] Economic Commission for Latin America and the Caribbean (ECLAC). Social panorama of Latin America. Santiago: Cepal; 2020. Available from: https://www.cepal.org/en/publications/46688-social-panorama-latin-america-2020

[21] Ferreira P, Souza CTV, Santana CS, Nunes JA. Caring in times of COVID-19. Somatosphere: Science, Medicine, and Anthropology. 2020. Available from: http://somatosphere.net/2020/caring-in-times-of-covid-19.html/

[22] World Health Organization (WHO). Infection prevention and control guidance—(COVID-19). [S. l.]. 2020. Available from: https://www.who.int/westernpacific/emergencies/covid-19/technical-guidance/infection-preventioncontrol

[23] Gold MS, Sehayek D, Gabrielli S, Zhang X, McCusker C, Ben-Shoshan M. COVID-19 and comorbidities: A systematic review and meta-analysis. Postgraduate Medicine. 2020;**132**(8):749-755. DOI: 10.1080/00325481.2020.1786964

[24] World Health Organization (WHO). Food and nutrition tips during selfquarantine. [S. l.]. 2020. Available from: https://www.euro.who.int/en/healthtopics/health-emergencies/coronavirus-covid-19/technical-guidance/food-andnutrition-tips-during-self-quarantine.2020

[25] Brazil Ministry of Health. Health Surveillance Secretariat. Health Care Secretariat. National Health Promotion Policy/Ministry of Health, Health Surveillance Secretariat, Health Care Secretariat. 3rd ed. Brasília: Ministry of Health; 2010

Chapter 2

Perspective Chapter: Digital Assistive Technologies

Vivian Vimarlund and Diana Zandi

Abstract

The use of digital technologies has been described as a facilitator integrating services and offering facilities to support individuals with impairments. In this chapter we identify level of advancement, trends, and challenges in the growing area of digital assistive technologies. Interview with experts and a literature search were performed. The outcomes of this study shown that the generic use and adoption of technologies involves complexity and changes in several aspects and, specifically, requires changes in the overall practice environment. However, the real challenge is not to identify technologies or to prioritize products, policies, or praxis, rather it is to build infrastructures, to match levels of maturity with products or services, and to reduce the technical, and socio-economic inefficiencies that constrain the further development of the area.

Keywords: digital assistive technologies (DAT), challenges, levels of advancement, infrastructure, socio-technical and socioeconomic issues

1. Introduction

About 15% of the world's population lives with some form of disability. One billion people need assistive technology to live healthy, productive, and independent lives, and to participate in education, the labor force, and civic life [1–4]. It is estimated that this number will double by 2050 [4, 5]. With a progressively aging population and the rapid spread of chronic diseases (e.g., osteoarthritis, diabetes, depression, obstructive pulmonary diseases, dementia etc.), as well as continuing improvements in the methodologies used to measure disability, the number of people living with some form of impairment will rapidly increase, in virtually all countries. To overcome differences based on social and structural factors in the delivery of services to individuals with impairments (the elderly and individuals with disabilities), there has been a significant acceleration over the past 50 years in the development and use of digital assistive technologies (DAT) that improve the well-being of individuals in need [4, 6]. Technologies such as intelligent systems, assistive robots, wearable sensors, have gained attention due to their capacity to create real-time services [7, 8]. In parallel, concepts such as smart homes, intelligent homes, assistive technology, welfare technology, and ambient assisted living have flourished and are used to index research and development contributions aimed at supporting activities or services that address the requirements of individuals with impairments. Further, the use of digital assistive technologies has been described as an enabler integrating services and facilities that support and connect individuals [8–15]. During the last two years, a series of action plans have been developed to accelerate the development of online services. Private and public organizations have been forced to become more system-oriented to increase the capacity of clients, service providers, and stakeholders to respond to challenges such as the COVID 19 pandemic [16].

2. Aim

In this chapter we identify level of advancement, trends, and challenges in the growing area of digital assistive technologies. The outputs of the study can contribute to identify progression and pre-requisites to achieve a sustainable evolution of the area.

3. Method

Data has been sampled in several steps and taken from different sources with the aim to achieve consistency in the outcomes. At the first step, we performed interviews with six experts representing: (i) the WHO, (ii) academic institutions or research centers, and (iii) interest groups belonging to international scientific associations with market connections, as well as representatives of interest organizations with the aim of discussing barriers, facilitators, and issues of relevance for the implementation and adoption of digital assistive technologies. The interviews lasted between 60 and 90 minutes, and all of them were performed between January and March 2021. The interviews followed a semi-structured format, with guiding questions being used to ensure that a consistent dataset was collected from each respondent. Detailed notes were taken during the interviews. A summary of the main issues discussed during the interview was given by the interviewer at the end of the interview with the aim of ascertaining that the interviewee had been correctly interpreted. The answers were then registered in tabular form to facilitate comparison between interviews. In the next step we performed a literature search to capture examples and to illustrate progression or innovation of emerging technologies in the area. The literature search was performed in an iterative manner. In contrast to a systematic review, the interactive process allowed us to summarize the findings of the literature and rapidly achieve a broad coverage of the field. The concepts of ambient assisted living, smart homes and assistive technologies were used to search examples of implemented or suggested technologies. The search for literature was entirely conducted using electronic databases such as: Science IEEE Xplore Digital Library (https://ieeexplore.ieee.org/Xplore/home.jsp); ACM Digital Library (https://dl.acm.org/); and Direct (https://www.sciencedirect.com/).Only peer-reviewed publications written in English that discussed issues related to one or more of: systems, devices, products, services, to support individuals with impairments were included. Articles aiming to resolve purely clinical situations were not included. We adapted a model developed in a previous study to capture maturity and levels of advancement of eHealth applications to group DAT examples [15]. The examples were then associated with some of the area they aimed to support (accessibility, connectedness, engagement, and/or efficiency) and to the functions to which they contribute: cognition and sensory functions, mobility, daily living, communication, education, recreation, and/or sport.

4. Results

The ways in which DAT can support individuals with impairments in the long run, and the expectations and challenges for the further and sustainable development and distribution of DAT, as expressed by experts, researchers, and representatives from interest organizations, are described in **Table 1**.

	Expectations	Challenges
WHO experts	Ability to monitor, follow up and support individuals with impairments at a distance	• Absence of individual-based information to further the development of services • Different rules, policies, laws, and praxis in different countries
	Give individuals the opportunity to be included in societal activities. For instance: education, the workforce, health and social care, and leisure time activities	• Different levels of ICT maturity in different regions and countries • Absence of infrastructure (social or technical)
	Access to DAT and to real-time information offered by the community	• Lack of connectivity • Absence of technical structures and virtual platforms • Social and political structures are different in different regions
	Market products (devices and applications) are becoming cheaper because of global competition.	• Technical, or assistive products do not face the same level of competition as other products, and the number of items sold is very small, which might not allow an economy of scale effect. • DAT products or services are still expensive for some groups of consumers (i.e., low-income versus high-income countries). • Willingness to pay and budget constrains can be influenced by individuals' age, gender, income, education, and/or where they live.
Researchers	Opportunity to offer digital services (i.e., eHealth services, or online educational services).	• Difficult to keep service providers up to date with technological advancements
	Opportunity to support individuals with impairments at distance while maintaining service quality	• Mismatch between state-of-the-art of the technology and organizational or individual capacity to buy, distribute, or use devices, products, or services.
	Preventing emergency situations and reducing the burden of health and social care	• Complex organizational barriers or absence of clear ownership of the issues related to assistive technology
	Allow individuals to live more independently and for longer at home	• Different levels of ICT maturity at both the provider and the customer level
	Personalization of services	• Individual-based data is not accessible

	Expectations	Challenges
	Possibility to offer assistive technologies and services worldwide	• Differences in the level of technological advancement in different regions • Major focus on technology rather than on issues related to the acceptance of DAT • Absence of networks to develop collaborative road maps
Representatives from interest organizations	Access to mainstream devices and services for individuals with impairments	• Difficult to scale products • Focus on innovative products rather than on how to stimulate a circular economy, or outlet of DAT • The user of the technology is frequently someone else (e.g., informal caregivers) not the single individual (end-user).
	Opportunity to develop a digital society and become connected	• Market dominance (few actors) • Absence of basic infrastructures in some regions (e.g., absence of electricity) • Absence of educational programs to train users and personnel

Table 1.
Expectations and challenges for further development of DAT: Opinions from experts, researchers, healthcare, and market representatives.

It is interesting to note that the mismatch between the rapid development of technology and the capacity to buy, use, and distribute products are mentioned by researchers as among the major issues for the sustainable distribution of DAT. It is also interesting to note that technology itself (type of devices, services, or technical solutions) is considered to play only a partial role in the integration of individuals into virtual worlds. Social barriers, and the absence of technical structures, or even basic structures, as well as the absence of clear ownership of DAT, and the absence of training programs for both users and suppliers, are mentioned by the respondents as major issues that need to be resolved before continuing to discuss the further development of DAT. An interesting observation is that none of the interviewees identified areas or types of services that could be developed globally, nor did they mention the customer and their preferences, or the importance of age, gender, culture, or willingness to change routines as major constraints for the acceptance of DAT. Some of the interviewees mentioned the importance of the market and the market dominance of some companies for the sustainable development and distribution of DAT.

In the next step we group examples of digital assistive technologies and illustrate trends, levels of technological advancement, and challenges. (See **Figure 1**).

Group 1: Diversity in the development of the infrastructure and distribution of digital assistive technology: Analog solutions and isolated technologies.

The contexts (regions or local communities) in which digital assistive technologies are implemented do not always have digital infrastructures in place that support the implementation and distribution of DAT, and no clear organization for

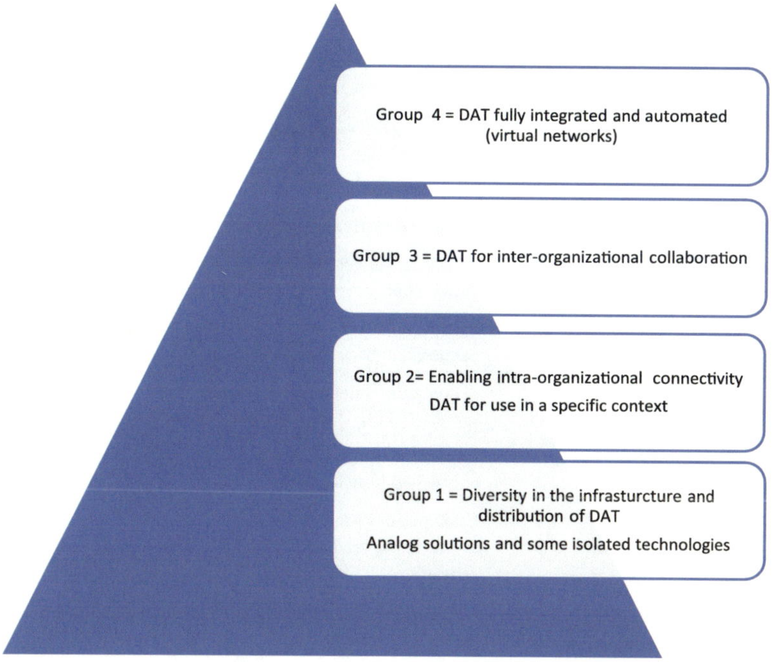

Figure 1.
Digital technology advancement, and pre-requisites. From diversity in the infrastructure to virtual networks (adapted from Vimarlund V., Kock S. 2016) [15].

the supply or distribution of services is in place. The accessibility of DAT cannot be guaranteed, and the use of products and services depends on socio-economic, technical, and cultural variables as well as geographical differences [14, 15, 17–27]. In the same context, it may be possible for some individuals to acquire or rent DAT devices or services, while others cannot. Issues related to the distribution of assistive technologies, in general, belong to different political actors and are not coordinated with the health or social care system. Basic phones with low functionality that primarily allow voice calls, SMS, are used as an alternative, in the absence of technical platforms, to access some services. Examples of products, devices, and technologies for this group are listed in **Table 2**.

Paradoxically, the main challenges at this level are not related to technology or technological advancements. The real challenges are: a) how to build platforms that provide solid and efficiently support to deliver products and services, b) how to build a roadmap that sustains the digital transformation needed to support the accessibility, and distribution of services, c) how to use simple available technologies, e.g. mobile phones to deliver basic DAT services, and d) how to develop an equitable and equal model that ensures security and performance and at the same time considers issues related to lifestyles, cultural differences, language differences, and d) how to motivate individuals to test and use DAT.

Group 2: Enabling intra-organizational connectivity for service transfer.

As countries advance in the development of their technical infrastructures, they make the Internet accessible to their citizens. DAT are mainly used to support the provision and delivery of services that facilitate one-way communication between one individual and one service provider. DAT are designed to address specific situations (e.g., to recognize actions or situations within the environment

Areas	Functions	Examples of products, devices, and services
Efficiency	Cognition and sensory functions	Conventional products to assist cognitive functions for planning and/or scheduling of services: • Memory devices and pill box reminders, alarms, etc. • Medication dispensing and management, rimers (time a person expends in the bath) • Sensory functions, e.g., spectacles, software for screen magnification and reading, hearing aids
Connectedness	Mobility	• Wheelchairs equipped with Bluetooth modules • Spinal orthotics and cervical collars equipped with dials to select the correct height setting
Accessibility	Daily living	• Adjustable Toilet chairs, diapers • Products for housing, work, and living environment or products for improvement and home modifications e.g., handrails, grab-bars, controlled lighting. • Basic phones for visually impaired individuals to make phone calls, access apps, read and send text messages and emails, set calendar reminders
Accessibility	Communication and education	• Voice and speech training devices • Braille apparatus and screen readers • Braille translator (software to translates electronic documents into Braille) • Audio format (to access and read information through hearing) • Screen-reading software (to allow people with low vision and the blind to convert text on a computer screen and in documents to synthetic speech)
Engagement	Recreation and sports	• Modified sports equipment to facilitate engagement in different leisure-time activities.

Table 2.
Examples of areas, functions, and products in group 1.

through monitoring or follow-up, or to detect and respond to potential emergencies), and to enable individuals to remain active, socially connected, and independent [15, 26–33] (see **Table 3**).

DAT applications for intra-organizational connectivity normally do not allow opportunities to interact or exchange information in real-time, but they do allow users to capture and accumulate real-time data. They have neither automation nor verification mechanisms. The main outcomes are related to reducing work overload and improving individual follow-up and monitoring. Information is transferred in a digital format, and individual recipients of services do not necessarily need to have a high level of ICT maturity and digital literacy. Investments in DAT are mainly made to reduce costly and time-consuming activities (e.g., ordering goods or medicines, searching for information), or to facilitate the management, monitoring, and follow-up of individuals. At the organizational level, DAT tend to reduce the number of unintentional errors, allows rapid and effective access to information (for the planning and distribution of resources), and enables the reallocation of time and resources (personal, administration for follow-up), organizational learning, and shorter lead times for decision-making. The socio-economic consequences of the implementation

Areas	Functions	Examples of products and services
Efficiency	Cognition and sensory functions	• Alarms to detect emergencies (e.g., falls at home) • Wearable sensors to detect movement (daily monitoring) or to monitor vital signs • Devices and sensors to support, follow up, and monitor individuals with cognitive impairments • Mobile or wearable devices for automatic translation between any languages in cases where pronunciation is unclear.
Connectedness	Mobility	• Devices or products to facilitate mobility and transport (e.g., wheelchairs connected to the internet) • Wheeled robots and/or devices that facilitate mobility • Voice recognition applications to search information and to facilitate accessibility to certain services such as transport GPS and telecommunication devices • Digital maps for pedestrians delivered to hand-held devices and smartphones
Accessibility	Daily living	• Consumer-oriented services, e.g., e-commerce alternatives to order foods and/or goods, medicines, or assistive technology products. • Digital assistants and navigation tools that provide assistance with audio support. . • Monitoring and reminding via electronic drug dispenser systems (electronic, pill or medicine dispenser systems with built in reminder)
Engagement	Communication, education, and recreation	• Screen readers to facilitate searching for and sharing information • Music apps, reality games to manage pain or for individuals with cerebral paralysis • e-books that can be uploaded and used at the individual level to facilitate the acquisition of knowledge Graphical user interfaces, text editing software and telephony services

Table 3.
Examples of areas, functions, and products in group 2.

and use of DAT at this level are normally short-term results due to reductions in transaction costs[1] when administrative services can be rationalized.

Group 3: Inter-organizational collaboration.

In this group, DAT are used to allow two-sided communication, transfer information within and between different organizations, and to support across communication in real-time. DAT allow access to online services and interactivity of different networks. Legislation concerning personal data privacy (including data access, exchange, and

[1] The total costs of making a transaction, including the cost of planning, deciding, changing plans, resolving disputes, and after-sales. Transaction costs are one of the most significant factors in business operation and management.

Areas	Functions	Examples
Connectedness	Communication	• Text and voice messaging with pictures and speech • Mobile voice user interface and smartboards • Ontologies and user models for activity recognition and real-time monitoring
Engagement	Education and training	• Interactive learning systems that support individuals with disabilities to actively participate in educational programs • Autonomous learning-based example or semantic information • Virtual reality games to learn, train, and improve cognition
Accessibility	Daily living	• Voice assistance and virtual platforms • Video-based home monitoring and internet-based services (that connect individuals with different service providers) Digital services that allow access and interaction between providers and consumers of services (e.g., net doctors, legal services) Digital media to offer leisure-time activities at a distance Smart phones wirelessly connected to body sensors (to monitor health and clinical signs remotely (e.g., EKG, tests etc.)

Table 4.
Examples of areas, functions, and products in group 3.

ownership) as well as rules for data processing as well as certification principles are in place to make electronic transactions legitimate and to build trust among stakeholders.

Improvements in digital infrastructure, such as bandwidth or communication speed, information storage databases, web services and backups, standard formats for data transmission, data encryption, password protection in support of digitalizing information and data exchange are in place based on nationally adapted recommendations based on international guidelines [34]. DAT belonging to this group are characterized by a multiple organizational perspective and presupposes investments in assistive technologies that support cooperation, communication, and workflow as well as the production of services between several different suppliers and providers i.e., (health and social care organizations, business enterprises, non-profit organizations [35–41]. Consumers and users can access multi-home services (similar services produced and delivered by different producers) through platforms that allow interaction between suppliers and consumers. An issue related to DAT, however, is the asymmetry in the information that exists about the number of accredited companies, hybrid companies (companies that provide welfare services[2], communication, and even other services), service companies, or publicly owned companies, stakeholders, and entrepreneurs active in the market. Most of the applications and services are aimed at enhancing communication and socialization within a community. Smartphones are used as the most common virtual platform to access the services and information available on the Internet (see **Table 4**).

Many of the examples belonging to this group refer to devices that help their users to receive or capture information from the environment to actively participate in their

[2] Services that cover the basic well-being of individuals and society. They may be provided as a citizenship right and managed by governments and institutions or private actors. Welfare services usually strive to improve the situation of people in need.

Areas	Functions	Examples of DAT for automation of services
Efficiency	Environment	• Alerts for home • Energy management systems • Robotics, react to touch autonomous or mobile control of temperature etc. • Emergency response systems to monitor risks outside the home environment
Efficiency	Safety and security	• Home safety/security systems • Use of digital identity • Facial recognition to reduce the number of surfaces people need to touch • Fraud protection applications
Connectedness	Daily living	• Robots to assist individuals at home or in the workplace • 3D sound to facilitate real-time understanding of the type and position of objects • Transmission of parameters through wireless biomarkers • Companion robots for emotional and social support • Distributed systems with direct data links to laboratories for pattern analyses • Multimodal systems to generate data about vital signs from mobile apps
Accessibility	Communication and transport	• Portals for monitoring and access to online services • Machine learning and pattern recognition for communication and transport • Signaling products and voice interpretation services • Smart sidewalks
Engagement	Education and training	• Learning management systems • Virtual reality for training • Braille keyboard interfaces to guide blind people • Voice transcription apps
Engagement	Leisure time	• Virtual reality games to assist individuals with e.g., cognitive impairments • Interactive products for recreation, sport, culture, and leisure

Table 5.
Examples of areas, functions, and products in group 4.

local community. Digital assistive technology not only detects and reports incidents, but also prevent undesirable events problems with connecting assistive devices and products into everyday living contexts. Remote services are adopted to improve quality of life, support independence, and reallocate resources. New structures created using DAT enable the creation of integrated services to support daily life, avoid social isolation, and/or support social integration. Paradoxically, the main challenges are not related to the implementation of technological innovations or to their functional capacities, but to the willingness of users to engage, to the frequency of their use of services, devices or products, and governance of the same. Smartphones with adequate mobile coverage and connection to a mobile data network become a critical tool to enable people with impairments to live independent and socially connected lives when the technical infrastructure is not optimal. An important challenge for this group is that the relationship between cost and effectiveness is not necessarily either direct or linear [15].

Group 4: Virtual networks.

Digital technologies belonging to this group require the integration of systems through an infrastructure that sustains vertical integration. This group is characterized by an individually focused perspective and includes investments in DAT innovations in which the receiver (the individual) is an active participant and influences the demand and supply of services at all levels.

Automation of services has reached a mature level, where users are proactively involved in the services they use. At this level, services are transformed from a push to a pull format (they are demand-driven). The virtual context offers accessibility to services delivered by private business partnerships. Data repositories, interconnection, and interoperability, in addition to a reliable networking infrastructure, are in place. Different suppliers and various channels for the delivery of services ensure agile accessibility to services, systems, and devices. Smartphones, the most advanced category of mobile phones, contain many of the functionalities of a computer and allow users to download and operate applications to create customized functionalities and thus interact with, access, and use assistive products [41–48]. Examples of DAT are listed in **Table 5**.

DAT in this group presuppose the development of a 'virtual context', or 'virtual communities', access to the Internet, and connectivity. The paradox of this level is that the benefits derived from the implementation and use of DAT become easier to appreciate, although the technology is interwoven into all activities. DAT products and services belonging to this group are not intended to be standalone solutions. Home or living environments are equipped with information and computing technology and devices that are usually described as the Internet of Things. Consumers (users and workers) have a good level of ICT literacy and can handle, update, and manage their technology.

5. Conclusions

The area of DAT is expected to nurture the digital transformation worldwide, and in parallel to transform the entire value chain, addressing the emergence of infrastructures, new transaction mechanisms for improved trust and security, and the development of strategies to facilitate the distribution and accessibility of DAT. This, however, requires overcoming the challenge to integrate individual systems into networks of actors that bring together civil society, consumers, and producers who are willing to accept the social impacts of the new context [16, 48]. The rapid development of technology and the absence of technical structures, are, however, mentioned by the respondents as major issues that need to be resolved before continuing to discuss the further development of DAT.

This study shown that publications focused on the impacts of DAT emphasize on specific technologies and address generic problems. Furthermore, they are, in general, optimistic and assume that all individuals with impairments will be able to participate in society easily and actively if they use digital technologies. Most of the studies focus on a single functional disability or physical or mental limitation and discuss early proofs of concept or engage in a theoretical discussion about the effectiveness or contribution of DAT to resolve major socio-technical issues whereas the mainstream adoption of new technologies is not discussed [49, 50]. Most of the publications are related to diseases, geriatrics, healthcare, patient monitoring, artificial intelligence applications, epidemics, telerehabilitation, drug reposition, transport, or to the need to develop policies to ensure the accessibility to DAT. This makes the literature dispersed and fragmented rather than focused and with possibilities to replicate the outputs.

The classification of DAT we have suggested in this chapter, contributes to identifying pre-requisites that need to be fulfilled to achieve a sustainable progress from one step to another. The classification suggested shows further that when identifying the possibilities offered by DAT, it is important to consider issues such as existing infrastructures, maturing level, preferences as well as socio-technical and economic issues. This study demonstrates also, that when opening the 'black box' of DAT, there are several elements and challenges that the global community needs to resolve. Many questions remain to be answered. For instance, it is not yet known whether the COVID 19 pandemic will change patterns of interaction and communication in the long term. As we continue to adapt to the "new" normal of increased digitalization, the time has come for digital technology providers to continue to work closely with the four pillars of society to develop long-term solutions to bridge the digital gap. In future studies it will be necessary to discuss how patters of interactions and communications will change and what is needed to move from one phase to another in parallel to technological innovations which require a flexible strategy to achieve sustainability in the area.

Acknowledgements

This work has been supported by the WHO through the project "Digital assistive technologies" 2020.

Author details

Vivian Vimarlund[1,2*] and Diana Zandi[3]

1 Department of Computer and Information Science (IDA), Linköping University, Linköping, Sweden

2 Co-chair WG Ambient Assisted Living, IMIA

3 MScEE World Health Organization WHO, Geneva, Switzerland

*Address all correspondence to: vivian.vimarlund@liu.se

References

[1] WHO. The International Classification of Functioning, Disability and Health (ICF). Geneva: World Health Organization; 2001. Available from: https://unstats.un.org/unsd/demographic-social/meetings/2017/oman--disability-measurement-and-statistics/Session%205/UNSD_1.pdf

[2] Mort M, Milligan C, Roberts C. Chapter 1 healthcare at home? In: Ageing, Technology, and Home Care: New Actors, New Responsibilities. Paris: Presses des Mines; 2014. DOI: 10.4000/books.pressesmines1492

[3] United Nations, Department of Economic and Social Affairs, Population Division. World Population Ageing. 2015. (ST/ESA/SER.A/390)

[4] Blackman S, Matlo C, Bobrovitskiy C, Waldoch A, Fang ML, Jackson P, et al. Ambient assisted living technologies for aging well: A scoping review. Journal of Intelligent Systems. 2016;**25**(1):55-69

[5] WHO. World Report on Disability. Geneva: World Health Organization; 2011. ISBN: 9789241564182

[6] Foley A, Ferri BA. Technology for people, not disabilities: Ensuring access and inclusion. Journal of Research in Special Educational Needs. 2012;**12**(4):192-200. DOI: 10.1111/j.1471-3802.2011.01230.x

[7] Shengzhi W et al. Technology to support aging in place: Older adults' perspectives. Healthcare. 2019;**7**(2):60. DOI: 10.3390/healthcare7020060

[8] Vimarlund V, Borycki E, Kushniruk A, Avenberg K. Ambient assisted living: Identifying new challenges and needs for digital technologies and service innovation. IMIA Yearbook of Medical Informatics. 2021:16-34

[9] WHO. Policy Brief: Access to Assistive Technology. Geneva: World Health Organization; 2021 Available from: https://www.who.int/publications/i/item/978-92-4-000504-4

[10] United Nations Systems. A Shared United Nations System: Framework for Action Leaving No One behind. Equality and Non-Discrimination at the Heart of Sustainable Development. New York: United Nations; 2017 Available from: https://unsdg.un.org/2030-agenda/universal-values/leave-no-one-behind

[11] WHO. WHO Global Disability Action Plan 2014-2021. Better Health for all People with Disability. Action Plan 2014-2021. Geneva: WHO; 2015

[12] WHO. Global Cooperation on Assistive Technology (GATE). 2018. Available from: https://www.who.int/news-room/feature-stories/detail/global-cooperation-on-assistive-technology-(gate)

[13] Manzoor M, Vimarlund V. Digital technologies for social inclusion of individuals with disabilities. Health and Technology. 2018;**8**(5):377-390

[14] Webster J, Watson R. Analyzing the past to prepare for the future: Writing a literature review, MIS Quarterly. 2006;2: pp. xiii-xxiii

[15] Vimarlund V, Koch S. Identifying where the values come from IT-innovations in health and social care. Intelligent Information Management. 2012;**4**:296-308. Available from: https://www.researchgate.net/publication/232743185

[16] Smith E et al. Assistive technology use and provision during COVID-19: Results from a rapid global survey. International Journal of Health Policy and Management. 2020;**10**:1-10. DOI: 34172/ijhpm.2020.210

[17] Turing A. Can machines think? AI Magazine. 1992;**13**:2

[18] European Commission. Independent High-Level Expert Group on Artificial Intelligence. Set up by the European Commission. A Definition of AI: Main Capabilities and Disciplines. Directorate. General for Communications Networks, Content and Technology. Brussel: European Commission; 2019. Available from: https://digital-strategy.ec.europa.eu/en/library/definition-artificial-intelligence-main-capabilities-and-scientific-disciplines

[19] European Parliament. The Internet of Things Opportunities and Challenges, Briefing. European Union; 2015. Available from: http://www.eprs.ep.parl.union.eu (intranet)

[20] VanGrootven B, van Achterberg T. The European Union's ambient and assisted living. Joint programme. An evaluation of its impact on population health and well-being. Health Informatics Journal. 2016;**25**:27-40. DOI: 10.1177/1460458216683535

[21] Ramirez-Hernandez D, Stolwyk RJ, Chapman J, Dana WD. The experience and acceptability of smartphone reminder app training for people with acquired brain injury: A mixed methods study. Neuropsychological Rehabilitation. 2021;**2021**:1-28

[22] Pinard S, Bottari C, Laliberté C, Pigot H, Olivare M, Couture M, et al. Design and usability evaluation of COOK, an assistive technology for meal preparation for persons with severe TBI. Disability and Rehabilitation Assistive Technology. 2021;**16**(7):1-15

[23] Jamwal R, Callaway L, Farnworth L, Winkler DI. Electronic assistive technology use in Australian shared supported accommodation: Rates and user characteristics. Disability and Rehabilitation Assistive Technology. 2018;**13**(7):634-640

[24] Roopa M, Pattar S, Buyya R, et al. Social internet of things (SIoT): Foundations, thrust areas, systematic review and future directions. Computer Communications. 2019;**139**:32-57

[25] Radhhal M, Mirna AM, Ibrahim H. Health of humans and machines in a common perspective. Procedia Computer Science. 2020;**177**:415-422

[26] Rector K. Enchancing accessibility and engagement for those with disabilities. IEEE Pervasive Computing. 2018;**17**:9-12

[27] Weakley A, Tam JW, Van Son C, Schmitter-Edgecombe M. Effectiveness of a video-based aging services technology education program for health care professionals. Gerontology & Geriatrics Education. 2019;**40**(3):339-356

[28] Gagnon-Roy M, Bier N, Couture M, Giroux S, Pigot H, Zarshenas S, et al. Facilitators and obstacles to the use of a cognitive orthosis for meal preparation within the homes of adults with a moderate to severe traumatic brain injury: Informal caregivers and health-care professionals' perspectives. Assistive Technology. 2021;**4**:1-8

[29] Jamieson M, Cullen B, Lennon M, Brewster S, Evans J. Designing ApplTree: Usable scheduling software for people with cognitive impairments. Disability and Rehabilitation: Assistive Technology. 2020:1-11. DOI: 10.1080/17483107.2020.1785560

[30] Paunov C, Planes-Satorra S. What Future for Science Technology and Innovation after Covid-19? OECD Science, Technology and Industry Policy Papers. Paris: OECD Publishing; 2021 no 107. Rosemann M. Kowalielewicz M, Dootson P, Digital strategy of the future 2021. PWE Chair in. Paris: OECD Publishing;

[31] World Intellectual Property Organization. Technology Assistive Technology. Geneva, Switzerland: Trends; 2021

[32] Nordic Centre for Welfare and Social Issues Welfare Technology. 2010. Available from: www.nordicwelfare.org

[33] UNCTAD. Technology and Innovation Report 2021. Catching Technological Waves Innovation with Equity. Geneva, Switzerland: UNCTAD; 2021

[34] EU Fostering a European approach to Artificial Intelligence. Brussels 21, 4, 2021, Com (2021) 205 final

[35] Ambient Assisted Living & Smart Home Market Research Report by Product (Energy Management System, Entertainment Control, HVAC Control, and Security & Access Control), by Service (Customization & Renovation and Installation & Repair Service) - Global Forecast to 2025 - Cumulative Impact of COVID-19. Available from: https://www.reportlinker.com/p06025416/Ambient-Assisted-Living-Smart-Home-Market-Research-Report-by-Product-by-Service-Global-Forecast-to-Cumulative-Impact-of-COVID-19.html?utm_source=GNW

[36] Baert S, Lippens L, Moens E, Weytjens J, Sterkens P. The COVID 19 Crisis and Telework. A Research Survey on Experiences, Expectations, and Hopes. Global Labor Organization Discussion Paper N 532; Faculty of Economics and Business Administration. Ghent: Ghent University; 2020

[37] Chowdhury P, Paul SK, Kaisar S, Moktadir A. COVID-19 pandemic related supply chain studies: A systematic review. Transportation Research Part E: Logistics and Transportation Review. 2021;**148**:102271

[38] Chadoulos S, Koutsopoulos I, Polyzos G. Mobile apps meet the smart energy grid: A survey on consumer engagement and machine learning applications. IEEE Access. 2020;**8**:2169-3536. DOI: 10.1109/ACCESS.2020.3042758

[39] Alam MR, Reaz MB, Mohd Ali MA. A review of smart homes- past, present, and future. IEEE Transactions on Systems Man and Cybernetics Part C. 2020;**42**(6):1190-1203. DOI: 10.1109/TSMCC.2012.2189204

[40] Kim MJ, Cho ME, Jun HJ. Developing design solutions for smart homes through user-centered scenarios. Frontiers in Psychology. 2020;**11**:335. DOI: 10.3389/fpsyg.2020.0033

[41] Serrenho T, Bertoldi P. Smart Home and Appliances: State of the Art. Energy, Communications, Protocols, Standard. Luxembourg: European Union; 2019

[42] Cozza M, Crevani L, Hallin A, Schaeffer J. Future ageing: Welfare technology practices for our future older selves. Futures. 2019;**109**:117-129

[43] Budd J, Miller BS, Manning EM, Lampos V, Zhuang M, Edelstrin M, et al. Digital technologies in the public health response to COVID 19. Nature Medicine. 2020;**26**:1-10

[44] Ericsson LM. Consumer & IndustryLab. Keeping Consumers

Connected in a COVID-19. Ericsson Consumer & IndustryLab; 2020. Available from: https://www.ericsson.com/en/mobility-report/articles/connected-consumers-getting-through-the-pandemic

[45] Ejaz WM, Basharat M, Saadat S, Khattak AM, Naeem M, Anpalagan A. Earning paradigms for communication and computing technologies in IoT systems. Computer Communications. 2020;**153**:11-25

[46] Drigas A. Special education and ICTs. International Journal of Emerging Technologies in Learning. 2013;**8**(2):41-47. DOI: 10.3991/ijet.v8i2.2514

[47] Zhou Y, Rehman RZU, Hansen C, Maetzler W, Del Din S, Rochester L, et al. Classification of neurological patients to identify fallers based on spatial-temporal gait characteristics measured by a wearable device. Sensors. 2020;**20**(15):4098. DOI: 10.3390/s20154098

[48] Holzinger A, Errath M, Searle G, Thurnher B, Slany W. From extreme programming and usability engineering to extreme usability in software engineering education. In: 29th Annual International Computer Software and Applications Conference. Vol. 2. *COMPSAC IEEE*; IEEE; 2005. pp. 169-172

[49] Abdi S, de Witte L, Hawley M. Emerging technologies with potential care and support applications for older people: Review of gray literature. JMIR Aging. 2020;**3**(2):e17286. DOI: 10.2196/17286

[50] World Health Organization. Global perspectives on assistive technology. Proceedings of the GReaT Consultation, Vol 2. Geneva, Switzerland: WHO; August 2019;**2**:22-23

Section 2

Health Promotion Practices

Chapter 3

'Lenzgesund': A Long-Term Community Health Promotion Programme in a Deprived Neighbourhood and Its Evaluation

Alf Trojan

Abstract

The contribution will present a highly visible health promotion programme in a deprived urban neighbourhood, initiated in 2004 by the health authority of the Hamburgian district Eimsbüttel. Its focus was on capacity building in cooperation with local actors/parties and residents. During 2005 and 2017, the programme, called 'Lenzgesund', was researched by a team of the Institute of Medical Sociology. The research aimed at giving feedback to the actors about how well they achieved their goals. For this purpose, we had to develop and test new approaches to evaluation. KEQ (Kapazitätsentwicklung im Quartier/capacity building in residential quarters/ neighbourhoods) is the acronym of a newly developed questionnaire for measuring community capacities being considered as relevant for health. KEQ can be seen as an intermediate outcome parameter for health promotion programmes and activities on the community level. Another innovative approach to evaluation was an audit of the programme through experts from outside Hamburg in order to have a more neutral external view. The first paragraphs will present the practical programme and its development in phases from 2004 to 2012. In the second part, we will give a short account of the two main approaches to long-term evaluation of the programme.

Keywords: health promotion, prevention, evaluation, capacity building, audit

1. Introduction

A frequent criticism of health education interventions (nowadays usually also referred to as health promotion measures) relates to the fact that merely behavioural changes in individuals are encouraged and that the mostly minor successes are not sustainable. The Ottawa Charter for Health Promotion (1986) [1] proposed a new focus: emphasis should be placed on changing relationships, making structural improvements at a local level and the participation of residents. This concept was later defined as Healthy Public Policies [2] and has proven to be at least partially effective in exemplary studies [3] as well as in a more recent review [4].

The following is a report about a community health promotion programme in this sense. The first part of the article (sections 2–4) deals with the 'Lenzgesund' action programme (named after the neighbourhood's name of 'Lenzsiedlung') implemented by the public health authority in one of the larger boroughs of Hamburg. The second part (sections 5–8) consists of an account of accompanying research from a total of three projects and the action programme's evaluation by the Institute of Medical Sociology at the University Medical Center Hamburg-Eppendorf.

The detailed presentation of this programme and its accompanying research results is legitimised mostly by the fact that it won the Academy's quality award for public health in 2014 [5].

2. Start of the Lenzgesund prevention programme

In the Hamburg borough of Eimsbüttel, the local public health authority began its work on health promotion and reporting measures in the second half of the 1990s. After a series of projects designed 'top-down' during the initial phase (including school vaccination projects and regular information events on health and environmental issues), the public health authority then began its first small-scale, low-threshold and more participatory health promotion measures in 2001 in the Lenzsiedlung of the Hamburg borough of Eimsbüttel.

This is a high-rise housing estate with 3000 residents in social housing. It is worth highlighting that the proportion of children and adolescents, migrants, single parents and recipients of social security is well above the Hamburg average ([6], p. 50ff).

The measures were developed to target young families in particular. Since the public health authority had no human resources and only very few material resources for health promotion measures according to the establishment plan, it needed to acquire cooperation partners and to develop additional financial resources for this project.

In October 2003, the public health authority invited in institutions from the areas of social affairs, child and family support, education and health care who were working in or on behalf of the Lenzsiedlung. It suggested setting up a round table to develop health promotion measures or to increase their effectiveness by cooperating and networking. The presence of a permanent practice partner on location in the form of the neighbourhood association 'Lenzsiedlung e.V. – Association for Children, Youth and Community' [7] was highly beneficial.

In November 2003, the Institute of Medical Sociology (IMS) at the University Medical Center Hamburg-Eppendorf and the public health authority Eimsbüttel agreed to collaborate on a research project into health promotion through the formation of structures to develop capacities in the Lenzsiedlung. In 2004, for the IMS' funding application to the Federal Ministry of Education and Research, the public health authority developed a detailed 'Preliminary Action Concept' for a planned project called the 'Lenzgesund Prevention Programme – Networked Early Support Measures for Pregnancy, Birth and the First Years of Life' [8].

Once the research project had been approved, preliminary action and research concepts were presented to the round table in January 2005, and the participants were invited to jointly implement and further develop the prevention programme, which met with a positive response.

Even though Lenzgesund only had access to material resources in the middle four-digit range in addition to a grant to finance a family midwifery offer and to provide eight working hours per week for planning and organisation, it was nevertheless an ambitious project for the borough at the time, which increased its importance and the 'health promotion' task's organisational embedding in the authority.

The regular feedback the research group presented to the round table strengthened the latter's function and cohesion and promoted the role documentation, evaluation and quality development played as part of the practical work.

3. Main features of the Lenzgesund prevention programme

The method chosen in the Lenzsiedlung can be characterised as a participation-oriented 'bottom-up' approach to neighbourhood-related *health promotion* and is characterised by the following design elements: health promotion is primarily designed *within a residential* area by parties who are *already active there* and is primarily aimed at the area's residents. *Offers from external providers,* for example prevention courses, in individual cases also those partially subsidised by health insurance companies or advisory services, are brought into the neighbourhood. The offers are made visible to all residents via internal *communication channels within the neighbourhood.* In the same way, the providers receive feedback relatively quickly for the offers' *needs-based further development* and expansion. *Communication and cooperation* form the core of neighbourhood-focused health promotion. To this end, the *'permanent' presence* of a contact person as well as of a coordinator and a cooperation and coordination committee are important.

The prevention programme's overriding aim was to promote health and to strengthen the social opportunities available to the Lenzsiedlung's residents. The development of community capacities played a crucial role (see below for their definition and measurement).

The preliminary action plan presented by the public health authority ([9], p. 71ff) defined the following 9 or 11 fields of action in which the abovementioned goals should be pursued:

- Birth preparation
- Pregnancy and parenthood of minors
- Support after birth and during the first year of life
- Vaccination
- Early intervention
- Dental health care
- Nutrition
- Exercise
- Health action competence/Health literacy

For each field of action goals, target groups, the initial situation, offers, opportunities to create structures, possible cooperation partners as well as success parameters and measurement methods were presented. Despite this detailed formulation, the preliminary action plan was not understood as an agenda that had to be implemented 1:1 but was rather intended as a 'powerful impact' that should give potential cooperation partners a decisive impetus for action.

4. Implementation and further development of Lenzgesund

The health promotion measures' development in the Lenzsiedlung, the timing of which did not entirely overlap that of the prevention programme, can be broken down into four major phases that had different 'development tasks', which we will briefly outline below.

2001–2003 Gaining a foothold in the neighbourhood

The phase was characterised by the planning, implementation and evaluation of initial offers and the establishment of local communication.

One of the offers was an external consultation hour for the borough's advisory service for mothers, which was, however, discontinued after 2 years due to a lack of response. With 16 events in 2 years, the 'Health talks for women by women' were strongly geared to the needs of migrant women both in terms of content and methods used. These were very well received. From autumn 2002 onwards, it became possible to employ a family midwife in the Lenzsiedlung who not only provided noticeable support for the neighbourhood's young families but was also considered by other institutions as an important addition to their own offers and who thereby prepared the basis for cooperation. This development ultimately led to the establishment of a 'Health Round Table' in the autumn of 2003.

2004–2010 Growth through cooperation

The topic of this phase was the development of a cooperative working structure and linked to it the offer's quantitative and qualitative strengthening.

The round table, which included youth welfare institutions, day-care centres, schools, the borough's administration and borough politicians as well as GP surgeries, pharmacies and other health care providers, initially dealt with collegial advice on current offers and the initiation of smaller projects such as a (multilingual) orientation guide on how to access health care services.

At the beginning of the cooperation, the start of the prevention programme and its scientific supervision in 2005 created new, activating impulses. In the months and years that followed, various parties/institutions developed further health promotion offers for the neighbourhood, including the 'baby driver's license' (a series of seminars for parents-to-be), a back training programme, the violence-prevention exercise programme Fit & Peaceful, the psychomotoric exercise programme, the 'health scout' (a contact centre that mediates between residents and the neighbourhood's official authorities), thematic speaking courses and the Zahn-Lenz dental-health campaign ([6], p. 182ff).

The round table met three times a year. In addition to reports from practical settings, specialist inputs and feedback from the accompanying research, at longer intervals it also reflected on the quality of its own way of operating and, if needed, adapted the programme to the changing situations in the neighbourhood.

2010–2012 Increased embedding

Increasingly, health promotion measures were incorporated into the offer profile of the local facilities and into the residents' range of expectations and even actions.

Starting in autumn 2009, the Lenzsiedlung association increasingly organised its own offers such as nutrition and exercise courses, swimming courses for female migrants and information events about, for example, breast cancer prevention and mental health.

Participants from previous events actively enquired about other offers, for example swimming courses or application-oriented language courses and became involved in organising them. Other residents began to develop their own offers such as dance classes for girls or boxing training for various target groups and have been managing these successfully for years.

2012 onwards Stabilisation

In mid-2012, the Eimsbüttel district office, two local housing associations and the Lenzsiedlung association prepared an agreement to secure the continuation and further development of important offers for the period after the prevention programme and neighbourhood's development would end. This included annual funds provided by the two housing companies in the low five-digit range, and the district office provided supporting work capacities as well as a disposition fund amounting to € 4000 per annum. This agreement was concluded in early 2013.

At this point in time, as declared at the beginning of its involvement in the neighbourhood, the public health authority had withdrawn from its role as initiator, moderator and organiser but at the same time pledged further support for health promotion measures. Some of the tasks previously performed by the round table, which was also dissolved in mid-2012, were integrated into two other local bodies.

When the formal prevention programme ended in mid-2012, health promotion in the Lenzsiedlung was at a quantitatively and qualitatively impressive stage of development. Various aspects of the situation which had been achieved by then indicated that the essential 'achievements' of 8 years of structured neighbourhood-related health promotion would continue to exist beyond 2012, and constructive further development seemed possible [6].

The following sections of this report investigate the extent to which the expectations for the sustainable embedding of the health promotion measures have been realised. Section 5 provides an overview of the three research phases or projects. Sections 6 and 7 focus on the two most important evaluation approaches which were used to present and assess the ongoing developments following the prevention programme's final phase in 2012 up to the end of 2016. Finally, Section 8 briefly discusses the current situation and perspectives.

5. The research projects at a glance

In November 2003, about 2 years after the first as yet unsystematic activities were carried out in the Lenzsiedlung by the Eimsbüttel public health authority, initial contact was made with the Institute of Medical Sociology at the University Medical Center Hamburg-Eppendorf. In 2004, these led to the research group's first application for funding from the Federal Ministry of Education and Research and to the application's approval. In early 2005, formal research began.

5.1 Research project 1: Developing evaluation methods in a participatory manner

The first project's primary *aim* (2005–2008) was to develop and test methods for evaluating small-scale neighbourhood-related health promotion measures. The tests and feedback also contributed to the further development of the practical activities.

The project's initial, innovative thematic core was the development of a survey instrument: Structure formation or *capacity development ('Capacity Building') as an intermediate success parameter* was to be designed, operationalised and tested. While the concept had been received and accepted in Germany, it was being not applied and used for scientific work.

A secondary, thematic core of the research project focused on *indicators for small-scale health reporting*. However, we will not be dealing with this topic further in this article [6].

In detail, the *Institute of Medical Sociology's activities during the first project* from 2005 to 2008 were as follows:

- A survey of the municipal capacities available in the Lenzsiedlung at the following times 2002 (retrospectively), 2005 and 2008;
- Conducting of a resident survey on health offers and needs (February/March 2006);
- Neighbourhood-specific evaluation of the results of physical school entrance examinations and school dental examinations in the first- and fourth-year primary school children;
- Preparation of two 'neighbourhood diagnoses', i.e. small-scale health reports (October 2006 and October 2007);
- Accompanying research on individual interventions;
- Creation of the overview 'Who is who in Lenzgesund?' (October 2007).

Based on this successful cooperation, it was possible to achieve the approval of the second project and a continuation of the joint work.

5.2 Research project 2: Generate knowledge and practical aids

The rare possibility of the long-term evaluation of a socio-spatial prevention programme in a disadvantaged neighbourhood was to be exploited in the second project (2009–2012) by continuing with the evaluations. In addition to the evaluation, a second focal point was to test the transfer of both the practical approaches and methods of evaluation and quality development.

A so-called health team was formed as a participatory planning and steering committee for the evaluation procedures and innovative interventions, which alongside the Institute of Medical Sociology also included the Lenzsiedlung association, the Rauhe Haus Eimsbüttel and the public health authority as the programme's sponsors and organisers [6].

5.3 The focus: The KEQ [capacity development in the neighbourhood] instrument

The research group's focus was on the surveys about the development of community capacities in the neighbourhood supported by the KEQ instrument, the results of which were presented and discussed at the round table [8].

The KEQ was developed on the basis of international preliminary work [10] and was explicitly introduced by Walter and Schwartz in 2003 as a benefit dimension and target parameter for prevention and health promotion measures ([11], p. 206). More detailed information on this has been published elsewhere [12, 13].

The score of the instrument can range from 1 to 5 points. When the score goes up, we have improvements on the respective dimension, when it goes down, this shows a decline in achievements. The reliability of the five subscales of KEQ was checked using Cronbach's alpha and Spearman-Brown's split-half coefficient. The internal consistency ranges from 0.82 to 0.94 and is without exception satisfactory [12].

The KEQ questionnaire as well as supporting information and materials for carrying out, evaluating and documenting future surveys is freely accessible on the Institute of Medical Sociology's website [14] as well as on other Internet platforms [15].

5.4 Research project 3: Sustainability checks

The long-term evaluation was aimed primarily at the aspects of quality development and stabilisation and covered the years 2014–2017 [16].

In terms of content, the process of stabilising offers for neighbourhood-related health promotion following the end of the prevention programme in the summer of 2012 should be presented and checked using various evaluation approaches (for the approaches not presented here, see [17]).

The focus was still on the method we developed for assessing the 'capacity development in the neighbourhood (KEQ)', which we intended to make even more practice-friendly in design. Another focus was the testing of an audit procedure, which was supposed to complement the various internal evaluation views by providing an outside view. Reports about these two evaluation approaches follow below.

6. Evaluation of the capacity development in the neighbourhood (KEQ)

The KEQ instrument has been presented in detail elsewhere [12] and was last presented in an improved and abridged version [18]. It allowed us to compare the previous results from 2011 against two points in time after the programme had expired (2015 and 2017).

The results for the five capacity development dimensions observed in the Lenzsiedlung neighbourhood (KEQ) have been summarised in an overview network diagram (see **Figure 1**). Average point values per dimension are shown for the years 2011 (t3), 2015 (t4) and 2017 (t5), that is for the final phase and the stabilisation phase of the Lenzgesund prevention programme that took place after the summer of 2012.

As a result, the continued positive KEQ assessments in the fifth survey (t5) should be emphasised. This applies equally to all dimensions, whereby compared with the third survey (t3), after a short-term decline, improvements were again observed in the 'health promotion' dimension in particular (mean: 3.6 at t5 compared with 3.2 at t4). This confirms that the capacity development process continued during the

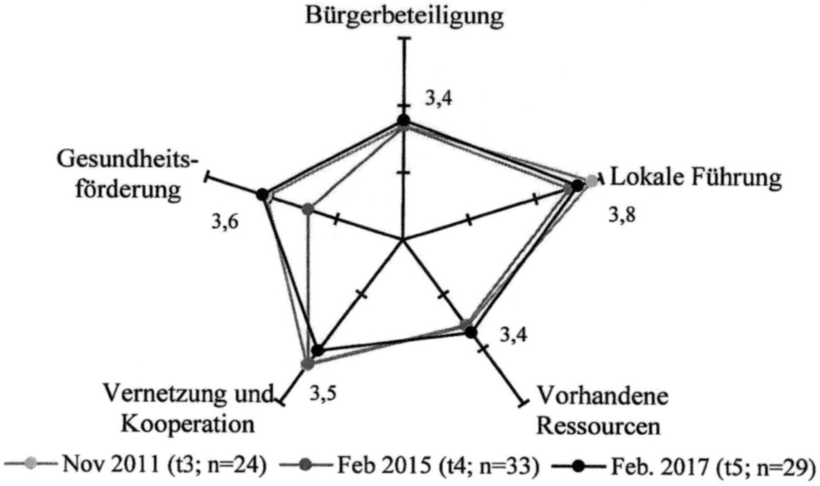

Figure 1.
An overview of the capacity development dimensions (mean values: 1 = worst, 5 = best value) (own illustration). Bürgerbeteiligung = public participation; Lokale Führung = local leadership; Vorhandene Ressourcen = available resources; Vernetzung und Kooperation = Networking/cooperation; Gesundheitsförderung = health promotion.

stabilisation phase. Despite the expiry of the official Lenzgesund prevention programme in 2012, a lot is obviously still going well and seems to be sustainable [18].

7. External evaluation *via* an audit

The KEQ instrument's aim is to allow for a quantitative survey of the community capacities. To do this, a significant number of people are usually needed who are both familiar with the community and who have the broadest possible general knowledge of the neighbourhood or district which extends beyond their respective specialised tasks. These respondents, however, represent an inside view of the outcome evaluation; in many cases they are also parties who are active in the neighbourhood at the same time. This leads to possible accusations that the local experts are too involved in the health promotion activities to give neutral answers, or, to put it even more blatantly: that the respondents would in fact be carrying out a self-evaluation and therefore evaluate the situation too positively.

To verify this, we organised a systematic review by five external experts and compared their assessments with the results of the local experts. Our procedure was closely based on an audit or the overlapping procedure of a peer review as it is practised in the medical field [19].

Table 1 summarises the document-based assessments of the first audit, i.e. the auditors' assessments for the years 2013/14 and relates them to the mean values from the KEQ survey of February 2015, which was also based on assessments for the years 2014/15. The auditors were of course unaware of the results of the KEQ survey. On average the auditors' assessments were more positive for all five dimensions. With a positive deviation of +0.1 to +0.9, they were, in some cases, significantly higher than the assessments of the local parties (column on the right of the table). This is particularly apparent for the dimensions 'Available resources' and 'Health promotion'.

	Reviews of the 5 auditors					Mean values in comparison		
	A1	A2	A3	A4	A5	A*	KEQ**	Δ***
Public participation	3.5	4.7	2.7	3.5	3.5	3.6	3.3	+0.3
Local leadership	4.5	4.5	3.5	4.0	3.0	3.9	3.8	+0.1
Available resources	3.7	4.6	3.2	4.0	4.0	3.9	3.3	+0.6
Networking/ cooperation	4.0	4.1	4.0	4.0	3.5	3.9	3.6	+0.3
Health promotion	4.1	4.5	3.8	4.0	4.0	4.1	3.2	+0.9

**External assessment by the auditors (A).*
***Self-assessment by local parties (KEQ).*
****Difference A–KEQ (Δ).*

Table 1.
External and self-assessments up to t4 (2015) in comparison (individual assessments and mean values).

The individual statements made by the auditors (A1–A5) show that their assessments were not homogeneous, rather in some cases they do clearly differ, which is explored and discussed in more detail elsewhere [16, 20]. In general, the comparison shows that the external auditors working based on the documents provided from the accompanying research made more positive assessments than those we received from the parties involved in the neighbourhood using KEQ. We explained this mainly by the fact that the parties' high expectations are often disappointed during the course of everyday experience, and they accordingly rate their successes low.

Despite our reluctance to generalise too quickly, we can say that for evaluations it is not always true that self-evaluations always result in the assessments being too positive; as in our case, the opposite can also be true, namely there can be an insufficient appreciation of one's own achievements [20].

8. Conclusion and outlook

Our cooperation with the parties of the Lensziedlung could just as easily be called practice-oriented *evaluation* research or evaluative *practice-oriented* research. It was always about a 'hybrid', namely the implementation of a 'model' programme in a disadvantaged neighbourhood on the one hand and the development of model evaluation approaches on the other. The integration of scientific and practical evidence production approaches was a guiding principle for the entire cooperation process (since 2004), that is for the joint efforts of practical application and research in the Lenzsiedlung. We are convinced that the work put into the Lenzsiedlung was and is sustainable.

In addition to the positive results of the evaluations, we can also rejoice in concrete decisions in recent times: on the basis of the Prevention Act in Germany and its implementation in Hamburg, it has been decided that municipal or neighbourhood-related health promotion should be financed and implemented jointly by the public health authorities and social insurance institutions. The first of these cooperation projects in Hamburg is entitled: 'Local Networking Centre for Health Promotion: Healthy in Eimsbüttel' and since August 2018 has been managing health promotion measures in two further neighbourhoods [21] (Eidelstedt and Schnelsen-Süd) based on the trials conducted in the Lenzsiedlung.

However, the experiences gained from the programme will also continue to bear fruit beyond Hamburg: since June 2018, 'Lenzgesund' has been presented as an inspiring example for the development of integrated municipal health strategies on the service pages of the nationwide Internet portal 'Partner Process Health for All' [22]. The programme is furthermore held up as a model of good practice in the second large practice portal for equal health opportunities [23].

Acknowledgements

I would like to thank my colleagues Christian Lorentz, Waldemar Süß and Stefan Nickel for the dedicated research work they have carried out over the many years of our three joint projects!
We thank the Federal Ministry of Research for funding the three projects:

1. BMBF research project 'Capacity building for prevention and health promotion among children and parents in a disadvantaged neighbourhood' (FKZ: 01 EL 0414), 2005–2008.

2. BMBF research project 'Long-term evaluation and transfer potential of the' Lenzgesund 'prevention programme – development of practical aids for interventions, evaluation and monitoring of participatory health promotion in disadvantaged neighbourhoods' (FKZ: 01 EL 0812), 2009–2012.

BMBF research project 'Long-term evaluation of complex interventions in neighbourhood-related health promotion and prevention measures – An investigation of community capacities ten years after the start of the Lenzgesund programme' (FKZ: 01 EL 1410), 2014–2017.
Last but not the least, we would like to thank the parties and residents of the Lenzsiedlung for their dedicated work towards the programme's practical implementation and during the accompanying research!

Conflict of interest

There is no conflict of interests.

Author details

Alf Trojan
Institute of Medical Sociology, University Medical Center Hamburg-Eppendorf, Hamburg, Germany

*Address all correspondence to: trojan@uke.de

References

[1] WHO. Ottawa Charter. 1986. Available from: https://www.euro.who.int/de/publications/policy-documents/ottawa-charter-for-health-promotion [Accessed: 20 November 2021]

[2] Evers A, Farrant W, Trojan A. Healthy Public Policy at the Local Level. Frankfurt/ M., Boulder/ Colorado: Campus/ Westview; 1990

[3] Plümer KD, Kennedy L, Trojan A. Evaluating the implementation of the WHO Healthy Cities Programme across Germany (1999-2002): How are we doing? Health Promotion International. 2010;**25**:342-354

[4] Nickel S, von dem Knesebeck O. Effectiveness of community-based health promotion interventions in urban areas: A systematic review. Journal of Community Health. 2020;**45**(2):419-434

[5] Steinbach E. Award: "Lenzgesund". Public Health Focus. 2015;**31**(1):4 [Internet]. Available from: https://www.akademie-oegw.de/fileadmin/customers-data/Blickpunkt/Blickpunkt_2015/Blickpunkt%202015_01.pdf Accessed: 20 November 2021

[6] Trojan A, Süß W, Lorentz C, Nickel S, Wolf K. Neighbourhood-Related Health Promotion Measures. Implementation and Evaluation of an Integrated Living Environment-Related Approach. Weinheim / Basel: Beltz Juventa; 2013

[7] Lenzsiedlung e.V., Project description [Internet]. Available from: https://www.lenzsiedlung.de/ [Accessed: 20 November 2021]

[8] Süß W, Trojan A. An integrated action plan as a structurally preventive approach in the social space: The socially oriented prevention program Lenzgesund in a disadvantaged district in Hamburg-Eimsbüttel. Journal of Public Health. 2012;**20**(2):203-207

[9] Trojan A, Süß W, Lorentz C, Nickel S, Wolf K. Neighbourhood-Related Health Promotion Measures. Implementation and Evaluation of an Integrated Living Environment-Related Approach. Weinheim/Basel: Beltz Juventa; 2013. p. 71ff

[10] Hawe P, King L, Noort M. Indicators to Help with Capacity Building in Health Promotion. Sidney: NSW Health; 2000

[11] Walter U, Schwartz FW. Prevention. In: Schwartz FW et al., editors. The Public Health Book. Health and Healthcare. Munich and Vienna: Urban & Fischer; 2003. pp. 189-214

[12] Nickel S, Süß W, Trojan A. Measuring community capacities with "KEQ": Psychometric tests results for a newly developed instrument for health promotion programs in Germany. In: Brown D, editor. Capacity Building: Planning, Programs and Prospects. New York: Nova Science Publisher; 2016. pp. 55-84

[13] Nickel S, Süß W, Lorentz L, Trojan A. Long-term evaluation of community health promotion: Using capacity building as an intermediate outcome measure. Public Health. 2018;**162**(9):9-15

[14] Project Description [Internet]. Available from: https://www.uke.de/kliniken-institute/institute/medizinischesoziologie/forschung/ag_gesundheit.html [Accessed: 20 November 2021]

[15] Project Description [Internet]. Available from: www.lzg.nrw.de, www.

in-form.de [Accessed: 20 November 2021]

[16] Nickel S, Lorentz C, Süß W, Wolf K, Trojan A. Quality Development and Stabilisation of Neighbourhood-Related Health Promotion Measures. The Example of the Hamburg Programme "Lenzgesund". Berlin: LIT-Verlag; 2019

[17] Lorentz C, Trojan A. Evaluative documentation of socio-spatial health promotion measures. Experiences from the Lenzsiedlung – proposal for a standard instrument. Blickpunkt ÖGD. 2021;**37**(2):5-5 [Internet]. Available from: https://www.akademie-oegw.de/fileadmin/customers-data/Blickpunkt/Blickpunkt_2021/Blickpunkt_02_21_Ansicht_PDF_final.pdf https://www.akademie-oegw.de/fileadmin/customers-data/aktuelles/Newsletter_06_2021/210103_Standarddokumentation_Gesundheitsfoerderung_Muster.pdf [Accessed: 20 November 2021

[18] Nickel S, Trojan A. Capacity development in the quarter (KEQ) – An instrument for the evaluation and quality development of neighbourhood-related health promotion measures. (Capacity building in the neighbourhood – an instrument for evaluation and quality development in community health promotion measures). Prevention and Health Promotion. 2021. DOI: 10.1007/s11553-021-00853-w [epub ahead]

[19] Sens B, Pietsch B, Fischer B, et al. Terms and concepts of quality and epidemiology. GMS Medical Informatics, Biometry and Epidemiology. 2018;**14**(1):Doc04. DOI: 10.3205/mibe000182 (freely available from: http://www.egms.de/en/journals/mibe/2018-14/mibe000182.shtml) [Accessed: 20 November 2021]

[20] Trojan A, Lorentz C, Süß W, Nickel S. Evaluation of community capacities by neighbourhood parties and external experts in comparison – Results of the auditing of health promotion activities in the Hamburg Lenzsiedlung. (Comparing Community Capacities by Local Actors and External Experts: An Audit of Health Promotion Activities in Lenzsiedlung, Hamburg) Public Health Service. DOI: 10.1055/a-1532-1911 [epub ahead]

[21] Project Description [Internet]. Available from: http://www.eidelstedt-mitte.de/projekte/koordinationsbausteingesundheit.html [Accessed: 20 November 2021]

[22] Project Description [Internet]. Available from: https://www.inforo.online/search?q=lenzgesund) [Accessed: 20 November 2021]

[23] Project Description [Internet]. Available from: https://www.gesundheitliche-chancengleichheit.de/good-practice/praeventionsprogramm-lenzgesund/ [Accessed: 20 November 2021]

Chapter 4

How to Support Health When Aging at a Place Called Second Home?

Annikki Arola

Abstract

Today, we live in a world where migration is a fact. Due to this, in this context, we have a group of persons who will age in a context that differs from their country of birth. It is important to identify the opportunities and obstacles that these persons face when they age in the context of migration. This chapter will highlight how aging is described and what it means to grow old in a migration context. What makes the life worth living? What creates meaning in everyday life when aging far away from "home"? One way to explore this is to see it from the perspective of health promotion and salutogenesis, where the meaning derives from the sense of coherence.

Keywords: health promotion, daily activities, salutogenesis, migration, old age, capability

1. Introduction

It is crucial to understand and broaden the view of health in everyday life among older persons aging in migrations. By doing so, it is possible to reveal how to promote health and enable the persons to have a sense of coherence and well-being, despite the fact that they are aging at a place that is not their origin home. Even if the older persons have been living in the host country for ages, the bond to their country of birth is tight. The connections to country of birth are an important part of the sense of well-being in daily life. Therefore, the everyday life in host country will always be experiences as the "second home."

The meaning of home is a complex phenomenon. It has a central place in every person's life since a lot of time is spent there. The concept of home and the meaning of it may vary between different persons, but mostly home is connected to feeling of safety, security, and relaxation. Home is place where many memories are kept, it could also be a place that reflects our identity. It is also a place that is connected to important and meaningful activities. Home is much more than an objective physical place. There is always an emotional dimension connected to home.

2. Aging and migration

We all get older, and the aging process is a normal part of life. The aging process can be described from different aspects such as physical aging, social aging, and psychological aging [1]. How the aging process continues is connected to heritage, environment, and the person's life style [2]. A concept often used in the area of aging is the concept of successful aging, which means to have the opportunity to engage in daily life, experience good health, seen from an individual perspective. Other important part is to have the possibility to be in charge over one's daily life [3]. This means that when a person has the possibility to continue to manage daily life by using one's own capacity, the life satisfaction will maintain even if the physical status declines.

The perspective and how we relate to aging and old persons are connected to cultural contexts with its values and norms. According to Fung [4], perspective on aging is influenced by the cultural differences in different countries. Most persons make sense of their life through the values and norms in the specific cultural context, and by that it will also create differences in how aging is perceived. For example, in some cultures, aging persons are respected due to their life experiences and older persons are considered as wise and prudent. In other cultures, aging is seen as a decline. Thus, the respect for older persons is lower, and older persons might be seen as nonproductive and a cost for healthcare services in the society. This kind of differences in how aging is perceived has an impact on aging in the context of migration. As persons age in migration, they have their original culture with them. At the same time, they have to adapt to the new environment and culture in the host country. How the person experiences the aging in the new context is dependent on how the person can interact with others, how they are treated, and if they have the possibility to continue to engage in important and meaningful activities, which they have performed in their country of birth. The experience and the response from the environment, and the possibility to find meaning in life, can be seen as important issues on how the person is able to create a sense of coherence, SOC, in everyday life.

3. The impact of migration on sense of coherence

Sense of coherence, SOC, can be described as a person's understanding of his or her situation in life [5]. According to Antonovsky, [6] SOC includes three parts, which promote SOC: comprehensibility, manageability, and meaningfulness. Comprehensibility relates to an assumption that things in one's daily life happens for a reason and that it is in some way predictable. For persons aging in migration, comprehensibility can mean that the person understands the things happening in daily life, understands external structures in society, which may affect daily life. For example, understanding how healthcare services work and how to contact the health service or any other authorities. Additionally, knowledge about the norms and understanding of cultural-related activities in host country may either decrease or increase the sense of comprehensibility.

The second part in SOC is the manageability, which means that the older person is confident in his or her skills and other resources needed to be able to cope in challenging situations in daily life. When aging, there will be decline in functioning, both physical functioning and psychological functioning. This will have an impact on the everyday life and the person's possibilities to cope with daily activities. Seen from a migration perspective, manageability can be negatively affected if the environment does not recognize the remaining resources the person has and which can be used to manage everyday life in host country. If the resources are not recognized, the resources are not fully utilized to support health. On the other hand, if the expectations from environment are too high in relation to person's capability, then it might cause a stress reaction and, in that way, have a negative impact on health [7]. The third part in SOC is meaningfulness, which means that the person finds life meaningful, can find a purpose in daily life, and that he or she is prepared and motivated to invest one's energy to cope with situations in daily life. Meaningfulness has also a cultural dimension since meaning derives from the signs and symbols in the culture [8]. Therefore, for older persons aging in migration, it might be difficult to find meaning in daily life if there are difficulties in interpreting these signs and symbols. All of the parts that build up the sense of coherence are vital for the possibility to experience health in daily life when aging in migration. Social and psychological factors, and also the cultural context, can be seen as cornerstones of a strong SOC. A strong SOC can diminish stress on physiological functions [9] and, by doing so, support experience of health in daily life.

The difference between having a strong SOC and a weak SOC lies in what kind of resources the person has and which can be used to meet the challenges in daily life. Antonovsky [6] calls these resources for General Resistant Resources, GRR. These GRRs can be induvial or resources in the environment, which can be used to combat the stressors or challenges in daily life.

4. Health among older persons in migration

Since the number of older persons aging in migration is expected to increase in the future, it is important to increase our understanding of how health in everyday life is experienced by persons who are aging in a country that is not their country of birth. Older persons are often described as a fragile group, who are particularly vulnerable to illness, have decline in functional capacity and difficulties in coping independently with daily life. A particularly vulnerable group are older foreign-born persons who are now aging in a country that is not their home of origin. Surveys that have been done among these people indicate that they have a weaker health status in comparison with older native-born persons in same age group [1, 4]. With this in mind, this group of older persons is described as a particularly vulnerable group. Efforts are needed to enable this group of older persons to maintain health in everyday life. The efforts should strive for supporting older persons to use and utilize the resources they have. These resources the person can use to create a meaningful and functioning everyday life and thus have a good life during old age. To be able to identify the personal resources and the older person's view of this, it is important to use a person-centered approach. This approach highlights the older persons' own perspective of health in daily life and builds the frame for health promotion. By doing so, it is possible for the persons to maintain or improve health when health is examined on the basis of quality of life, participation in activities, and a sense of meaning in everyday life.

5. Dimensions of meaning in daily activities

Yerxa [10] has highlighted the connection between health and engagement in activities. The World Federation of Occupational Therapy (WFOT) defines activities (occupations) as: "...the everyday activities that people do as individuals, in families and with communities to occupy time and bring meaning and purpose to life. Occupations include things people need to, want to and are expected to do" [11]. Daily activities are also recognized and named by the culture in which they are performed, and therefore, it can be assumed that the daily activities are formed by our cultural background [12]. The meaning and value in activities are strongly connected to the person's narrative and previous life. When reflecting on older immigrants, the value and meaning derive from their cultural background and in that sense the meaning in daily activities is also connected to this. For this reason, health in everyday life is supported when the older person can use his capacity in various types of activities in daily living, both routine tasks and other meaningful and engaging activities, which gives some kind of self-rewarded value to the person.

There is also a connection between health, meaning, and value in activities, and this meaning derives from different dimensions of activity. According to Wilcock [13], the meaning aspect is connected to the possibility to experience doing, being, becoming, and belonging in daily life. The experience of doing, being, becoming, and belonging is universal among human beings and an important part of the experience of health in everyday life [14]. This is interesting to reflect on from the perspective of SOC, in combination with migration and aging. Obviously, the doing part is tightly connected to manageability. This is because it refers to the concrete doing or performing activities. The experience of being able to engage in activities in daily life adds value into the experience of health and well-being [15–17]. Therefore, decline in functional skills may have negative impact on manageability. But if the functional limitations can be corrected by environmental adaptations or by health promotion interventions, it might be possible to perform the activity even in future. The relation between health and ability to manage and engage in activities includes all kinds of activities, both productive activities and leisure activities [18]. Characteristic of these activities is that there is a deep emotional aspect, they are performed with passion and are more than just routine activities. Additionally, these activities are absorbed with positive meaning [16, 17], and they should be self-initiated [19].

For persons aging in migration, the opportunities to perform self-initiated activities increase the experience of health in daily life. Other important aspect is the connection between activities and the person's sense of belonging. Additionally, when the activities are defined and named within a group where the person experiences inclusion and belonging, the meaning in the activity will be even more valuable and rewarding. When a person is a member of a group, and has social support, it can be assumed that the social environment will be a source for supporting both manageability and comprehensibility when aging in migration. Especially, the connections to a group with compatriots have been seen to have an important impact on the sense of well-being [20]. Other important part of being able to experience health is the possibility to have moments of relaxation. In the context of migration, it means to be able to have a daily life without too much stressors, which requires great efforts by the person. Situations that are not comprehensible or manageable create a stress reaction. This will have a negative impact on the sense of coherence in all its parts, but especially comprehensibility and meaningfulness. Consequently, then the person cannot see what point it is in daily life and the things that are happening around him. The person will then not have opportunities for just being, which is an important part of the balance in daily life. When a person has opportunity to relax and have moments of being, it will create time for the person to reflect on life and think about what the future brings and what the person will become [13]. For persons aging in migrations, these reflections might be scary because it is connected to uncertainty in how to manage everyday activities if being dependent on others. Research has shown that some of the thoughts have to do with the challenges to communicate with professional care givers. The concern is that what happens if the older person cannot express his or her needs and wishes due to lack of language skills? The concern has to do with the existential dimension of being a person instead of just an object who needs care [20, 21]. The point is that how does the older immigrant reflect on their own "becoming" in the future? This kind of worries may have a negative impact on sense of coherence, which will weaken the experience of health in daily life.

6. Daily activities and migration

Activities in daily living are often taken for granted, and we do not reflect on how decline, for example, decline in physical functions, may affect the possibility to perform daily activities independently. Different cultures may have different view of which daily activities are the important ones and how these activities should be conducted. For example, it might be that older immigrants have daily activities, which they are used to perform in a specific way, and which are meaningful. In situations where they need care from healthcare professionals, situations can occur where the professionals do not recognize the meaning dimension in the activity. In these situations, the value and meaning in activities will decrease, and there may be a disruption in daily activities [22, 23], which may affect the experience of health in daily life. In addition to physical functions, also the environment where the activities are performed will have an impact on how the person can manage the activities. The environment can be both the physical environment and the social environment. If there are hinders in the environment, it causes decreased possibility for the person to use the personal capacity. This can be related to the concept of capability [24] where the view of human beings is that every person is capable of managing daily life if the personal resources and external surrounding enable the person to use their ability. Robeyens [24] explains that there are different types conversion factors, which influence how the person is able to use the skills and resources he or she has. These conversion factors are connected to the person's skills and body functions, social norms, and environment. In the capability approach, the environment is described on different levels such as organizational level, which can be interpreted as the political level. There is also the community level, which may refer to healthcare organizations and community. So, it is crucial to create environment that supports the person to use the capability he or she has. Healthcare organization should be responsible for creating structures and services, which are understandable and which enable persons to use their own resources. By this, the person will be able to use one's capability and create a valuable and meaningful life. How this is realized depends on what real opportunities the person has to engage in those activities and doings, which are meaningful and valuable for the person. Reflecting on this, if the surrounding and healthcare system are difficult to grasp and understand for the older person, it will decrease the person's possibilities to use the capability needed to manage daily life. Lack of information or knowledge of the system will have a negative impact on person's comprehensibility. Consequently, it will have a negative impact on the sense of coherence, meaning, and life satisfaction in everyday life.

The basis for engagement in daily activities is the personal motivation [16] and also a personal freedom to choose what activities are valuable and worth investing energy in. The motivation to perform activities is also connected to the possibility to perform activities in a way that is familiar to the person. In other words, to be able to keep up the familiar routines in daily life. How activities are performed has also a cultural dimension. Different dimensions of a culture create meaning to our activities [25, 26]. So, when moving from one cultural context to other, it may affect the meaning in the activity. In migration context, this is visible when older persons want to continue to perform activities in the same way as before immigration. Then the daily routines and meaning aspect in activities could be remained and by that support the meaningful parts of SOC. Professionals working with older immigrants have expressed that activities that are familiar from the country of birth are important for the experience of health and also as a way to keep up one's connection to the country of birth [20].

7. Health promotion as means to support everyday life when aging in migration

The goal with health promotion is to empower persons to maintain or improve their health and well-being in everyday life [27]. The traditional way to support health has been based on a deficit model, meaning that the focus has been more on decline and illness than the health resources the person has. Antonovsky's [6] perspective, with health as a continuum instead of a dichotomy where health and disease are opposites, has been highlighted as a more useful way of defining health promotion. Eriksson and Lindström [28] have created a metaphor for this perspective, which they call for "Health in the river of life." This perspective highlights the importance of changing the perspective from the traditional view in medicine, where the focus is on care and treatment, to a more holistic perspective where the core is on prevention and promotion. A similar view has been highlighted by Morgan and Ziglio [27], and they have stated that in health promotion, more resources and research need to be focusing on health resources as a way to promote health. Morgan and Ziglio present a model they call for the Health Assets model. In this model, the resources that could be used to promote health include resources on individual level, group level, and communities, populations, and social systems. When using all these resources through cross-border activities, it is possible to utilize more capability resources for individuals. When it comes to resources, more attention should be on identifying the individual resources that older persons aging in migration have. To be able to identify these resources, we have to combine perspective of salutogenesis with a person-centered approach in health promotion. A salutogen perspective draws a picture of what kind of situations in everyday life have an impact on sense of coherence among older immigrants. Furthermore, with a person-centered approach, it is possible to identify these resources together with the older person, with the aim to enable a meaningful life in the context of migration. Thus, a possible way to enable and support health among older immigrants is to create person-centered health promotion programs. The starting point in a person-centered approach health promotion is the concrete situations where the person is at the moment. The goal for person-centered health promotion is to empower the person to utilize his or her capabilities, including the resources the person has. This means to use the person's previous experiences and potentials. The focus should be on those life tasks that the person perceives as important and meaningful from a personal level. In everyday life, this means that the person has the opportunity to engage in those everyday activities, which creates meaning and value in life. This will also support the sense of coherence in daily life. Research has shown that even if the SOC is quite stable later in life, it is possible to influence SOC by using person-centered health promotion intervention [29].

The core of the person-centered approach is to have the person in center and involve the person as an active partner in both planning and implementation of health promotion activities. In person-centered health promotion, the relationship is based on equal interest, understanding, and importance. It is important to have the focus on the whole person, to find a common ground but also to find realistic frame for the intervention. Thus, when planning for health promotion from the perspective of salutogenesis and migration, the starting point should be to encounter the person in his or her specific context. This means, to be able to create a relationship with the person, which creates a trustful situation. When doing so, it creates an opportunity to be familiar with the person's narrative. The narrative will reveal the range of valuable and meaningful activities in everyday life. The mapping of the narrative, in combination with an authentic dialog with the professionals, is a way to empower the person to actively take part and responsibility for health promotion activities. An authentic dialog builds up a trustful relationship with the person, and it creates a mutual understanding for the planned health promotion intervention. The person is then seen, heard, and respected. The intervention is based on cooperation and mutual understanding where the person is an equivalent partner in the situation. It creates opportunities for the person to reveal thoughts and fears about issues that have an impact on comprehensibility, manageability, and meaningfulness in everyday life. A person-centered approach to health promotion, as a mean to support sense of coherence, can be argued to be a suitable and useful approach when aiming to support health among older persons aging in migration. It will also move toward a view of positive health along the ease/disease continuum [6]. Additionally, it supports opportunities to create a meaningful everyday life and by that support a successful aging in the context of migration. Health promotion programs, which are designed and based on a person-centered approach, adapted to fit persons who are aging in migration, seem to support capability in daily life among older immigrants [30]. This kind of health promotion interventions can preferable be conducted as group interventions consisting of persons representing similar migration background. Promising results have been revealed on this concept [31]. When older persons with immigrant background have the possibility to come together and discuss challenges in daily life, they have peer support from each other. This is a resource that supports experience of health and well-being in everyday life.

8. Conclusion

It is necessary to take a holistic view of health when discussing health in everyday life among older persons aging in migration. This is because persons are a product of their past lives. The person's narrative will give guidance on what kind of everyday life the older person wishes for when aging at a place called second home. The daily life should consist of activities that give meaning to life. Additionally, the situations in daily life should be comprehensible and manageable. For this reason, an important part is the environment and context around the person. Structures in healthcare organizations, such as health promotion, should be based on a person-centered approach. In this way, the person's wishes can be the starting point for health promotion interventions. A person-centered approach in health promotion enables both respect for the person and utilize the person's capability. This is the base for supporting and creating a meaningful daily life in migration context. Humans are able to create a meaningful life after migration when the daily life includes parts from the person's life before migrating, in combination with the routines and activities developed in the host country during resettlement. This means that older persons aging in migration can, with their own actions and wishes, be actively involved in shaping their daily life even in the context of migration. In this way, the migration does not have to be a negative influence on the experience of health or have a negative impact on sense of coherence.

Acknowledgements

This work was supported by The Finnish Ministry of Education and Arcada University of Applied science within the project AI Driven Nordic Health and Welfare.

Conflict of interest

The author declares no conflict of interest.

Author details

Annikki Arola
Arcada UAS Institution of health and welfare, Helsinki, Finland

*Address all correspondence to: annikki.arola@arcada.fi

References

[1] Delin O. Gerontologi: Åldrande i Ett Biologiskt, Psykologiskt Och Socialt Perspektiv [Aging in a Biological, Psychological and Social Perspective]. Stockholm: Natur och Kultur; 2000. p. 320

[2] Wilhelmson K. Att åldras. [Aging]. In: Dahlin-Ivanoff S, editor. Livslots för seniorer [Life slots for seniors]. Vårdalinstitutet: University of Gothenburg; 2009. pp. 9-26

[3] Grimby A, Grimby G. Åldrandets Villkor. [Aging Conditions]. Lund: Studentlitteratur; 2001. p. 224

[4] Fung H. Aging in culture. The Gerontologist. 2013;**53**(3):369-377. DOI: 10.1093/geront/gnt024

[5] Krause N. Deriving sense of meaning in late life: An overlooked forum for the development of interdisciplinary theory. In: Bengtsson V, Settersten R, editors. Handbook of Theories of Aging. 2nd ed. New York: Springer Publishing Company, LCC; 2009. pp. 101-116

[6] Antonovsky A, Elfstadius M. Hälsans Mysterium. [Unraveling the Mystery of Health]. Stockholm: Natur och kultur; 2005. p. 271

[7] Slootjes J, Keuzenkamp S, Saharso S. The mechanisms behind the formation of a strong sense of coherence (SOC): The role of migration and integration. Scandinavian Journal of Psychology. 2017;**58**(6):571-580. DOI: 10.1111/sjop.12400

[8] Bruner J. Acts of Meaning. Cambridge: Harvard University Press; 1990. p. 208

[9] Nilsson B, Holmgren L, Stegmayr B, Westman G. Sense of coherence - stability over time and relation to health, disease, and psychosocial changes in a general population: A longitudinal study. Scandinavian Journal of Public Health. 2003;**31**(4):297-304. DOI: 10.1080/14034940210164920

[10] Yerxa E. Health and the human spirit for occupation. The American Journal of Occupational Therapy. 1998;**52**:412-418. DOI: 10.5014/ajot.52.6.412

[11] World Federation of Occupational therapy. About occupational therapy. Available from: https://wfot.org/about/about-occupational-therapy [Accessed: 24-01-2022]

[12] Law M, Polatajko H, Baptiste S, Townsend E. Core concepts of occupational therapy. In: Townsend E, editor. Enabling Occupation: An Occupational Therapy Perspective. Ottawa: Canadian Association of Occupational Therapists; 1997. pp. 29-56

[13] Wilcock A. Reflections on doing, being and becoming. Australian Occupational Therapy Journal. 1999;**46**(1):1-11

[14] Erlandsson L-K, Eklund M, Persson D. Occupational value and relationships to meaning and health: Elaborations of the ValMO-model. Scandinavian Journal of Occupational Therapy. 2011;**18**(1):72-80. DOI: org/10.3109/11038121003671619

[15] Hocking C. Contribution of occupation to health and well-being. In: Schell B, Gillen G, Scaffa M, Cohn E, editors. Willard and Spackman's Occupational Therapy. 12th ed. Philadelphia: Wolters Kluwer Health/Lippincott Williams & Wilkins cop; 2013

[16] Kielhofner G. Model of Human Occupation: Theory and Application. 4th ed. Baltimore: Lippincott Williams & Wilkins cop; 2008. p. 565

[17] Nilsson I, Fisher A. Evaluating leisure activities in the oldest old. Scandinavian Journal of Occupational Therapy. 2006;**13**(1):31-37

[18] Menec V. The relation between everyday activities and successful aging: A 6-year longitudinal study. The Journals of Gerontology: Series B. 2003;**58**(2):74-82. DOI: 10.1093/geronb/58.2.s74

[19] Kim M. Life satisfaction, acculturation, and leisure participation among older urban Korean immigrants. World Leisure Journal. 2000;**42**(2):28-40. DOI: org/10.1080/04419057.2000.9674184

[20] Mårtensson AL, Häggblom Kronlöf G. Viewing oneself as a capable person – Experiences of professionals working with older Finnish immigrants. Scandinavian Journal of Caring Sciences. 2017;**31**(4):759-767. DOI: 10.1111/scs.12395

[21] Arola L, Dellenborg L, Häggblom-Kronlöf G. Occupational perspective of health among persons ageing in the context of migration. Journal of Occupational Science. 2018;**25**(1):65-75. DOI: 10.1080/14427591.2017.1368411

[22] Gupta J, Sullivan C. The central role of occupation in the doing, being and belonging of immigrant women. Journal of Occupational Science. 2013;**20**(1):23-35. DOI: org/10.1080/14427591.2012.717499

[23] Wright-St Clair V, Nayar S. Older Asian immigrants' participation as cultural enfranchisement. Journal of Occupational Science. 2017;**24**(1):64-75. DOI: 10.1080/14427591.2016.1214168

[24] Robeyns I. The capability approach: A theoretical survey. Journal of Human Development. 2005;**6**(1):93-117. DOI: org/10.1080/146498805200034266

[25] Hasselkus B. The Meaning of Everyday Occupation. 2nd ed. Thorofare: SLACK Inc; 2011. p. 216

[26] Persson D. Aspects of Meaning in Everyday Occupations and its Relationships to Health-Related Factors [Thesis]. Lund: Lund University; 2001

[27] Morgan A, Ziglio E. Revitalising the evidence base for public health: An assets model. Promotion and Education. 2007;**14**(2):17-22. DOI: 10.1177/10253823070140020701x

[28] Eriksson M, Lindström B. A salutogenic interpretation of the Ottawa charter. Health Promotion International. 2008;**23**(2):190-199. DOI: 10.1093/heapro/dan014

[29] Arola L, Barenfeld E, Dahlin-Ivanoff S, Häggblom-Kronlöf G. Distribution and evaluation of sense of coherence among older immigrants before and after a health promotion intervention – Results from the RCT study promoting aging migrants' capability. Clinical Interventions in Aging. 2018;**13**:2317-2328. DOI: org/10.2147/CIA.S177791

[30] Lood Q, Häggblom-Kronlöf G, Dahlin-Ivanoff S. Health promotion programme design and efficacy in relation to ageing persons with culturally and linguistically diverse backgrounds: A systematic literature review and meta-analysus. BMC Health Services Research. 2015;**15**(1):560. DOI: 10.1186/s12913-015-1222-4

[31] Barenfeld E. How to support knowing and doing in promotion of health: lessons learned from the Promoting Aging Migrants' Capabilities program [thesis].2016. Gothenburg: Sahlgrenska Academy at University of Gothenburg. Available at http://hdl.handle.net/2077/47404 [Accessed: 24-01-2022]

Chapter 5

Building Competency for Health Promoting Schools Development in Resource-Limited Settings: Case Studies from South Africa

Joyce Mashamba, Suraya Mohamed, Peter Delobelle and Hans Onya

Abstract

This chapter outlines the development of two health promoting schools (HPS) programs in resource-limited settings in South Africa, informed by work from two PhD tracks and a round table discussion on core health promotion competencies. The chapter focuses on the development, implementation, and evaluation of a training program for HPS among high school educators in the Limpopo Province guided by an assessment of priority needs; and factors influencing HPS implementation in three secondary schools in Cape Town. The first case study focuses on training program objectives, learning outcomes, and critical cross-field outcomes related to introducing the concept of HPS, empowerment of educators to initiate and evaluate HPS program design, and implementation. The second case study focuses on the role of external actors and stakeholders in designing and implementing HPS in resource-limited settings and the barriers and enablers related to HPS capacity building. The findings are discussed with reference to the national context and international literature and the competencies needed to guarantee successful HPS program implementation.

Keywords: health promoting schools, settings approach, health promotion competencies, educators, stakeholders, case studies

1. Introduction

Health promotion in schools has progressed rapidly since its inception in the last century, expanding from a traditional approach of health education in schools to its conceptualization as the Settings Approach to Health Promoting Schools (HPS). The concept draws on the five priority action areas for health improvement outlined by the Ottawa Charter for Health Promotion [1] applied to the schools setting and was piloted in Europe in the early 1990s by the European Network of Health Promoting Schools (ENHPS), which is now present in more than 43 European countries in the region [2].

The concept involves a whole-of-school approach to conducting health promotion and education in school communities, by capitalizing on its organizational potential to foster physical, social–emotional and psychological conditions for health as well as improved educational outcomes, and has been defined as "a school that constantly strengthens its capacity as a safe and healthy setting for living, learning and working" [3]. The HPS approach and related whole-of-school approaches to health have been associated with considerable improvements in many domains of health, well-being, nutrition and functioning [4].

In South Africa, the HPS concept was introduced in 1994 and guidelines drafted to comprehensively address school health in an attempt to redress the imbalances of the past [5]. South Africa adopted the conceptual framework of the HPS Network focusing on the school environment, community involvement, policy development and health and social services. By 2006, schools in all nine provinces were identifying themselves as health promoting schools [6]. A review on HPS conducted by Mukoma and Flisher [7] suggested that schools could successfully implement HPS, but no evaluation of HPS in Africa could be found.

A School Health Policy and Implementation Guideline document developed by the National Department of Health provided guidance for the implementation of health promotion activities through the 2015–2019 National Health Promotion Policy and Strategy [8]. The strategy, however, did not detail the systematic approach prescribed by WHO for initiating HPS, pointing to a weakness in the implementation of HPS that can be attributed partly to the system itself and partly to the quality of HPS concept implementation. Research was warranted to identify the causes of these weaknesses and to intervene by developing, implementing, and evaluating HPS initiatives.

In 2018, WHO/UNESCO announced an initiative to make every school a "health-promoting school, which included a commitment to develop global standards and indicators for HPS and to support their implementation [9]. These global standards and indicators were designed to be used by all stakeholders involved in identifying, planning, funding, implementing, monitoring, and evaluating the HPS approach and are applicable to any whole-of-school approach to health [10]. According to WHO [9], the whole-school approach is thus "an approach which goes beyond the learning and teaching in the classroom to pervade all aspects of the life of a school".

Although the HPS approach was introduced more than 25 years ago and has been promoted worldwide, the objective of a fully embedded, sustainable HPS system has only been implemented and sustained at scale in few countries [11]. Even fewer have effected institutional changes to make health promotion an integrated, sustainable part of the education system. Experts identified the lack of systematic support, the limited resources and common understanding as major barriers to HPS intervention [11]. These challenges are more pronounced in resource–limited settings, including South Africa and other settings in the global South.

Inadequate competency on the part of school authorities has been identified as a leading cause of HPS not being implemented and sustained at scale, in particular in resource–limited settings [12]. Health promotion competency frameworks spell out these 'competencies', which were defined as a combination of attributes that enable individuals to perform a set of tasks to an appropriate standard, such as knowledge, abilities, skills and attitudes [9]. The development of the global health promotion workforce brought renewed interest in identifying competencies for effective health promotion practice and education [13].

With a view of building health promotion capacity and workforce development, the identification of competencies is an important strategy for developing consensus around key requirements for effective health promotion practice [13]. A competent workforce which has the necessary knowledge, skills, and abilities to translate policy, theory and research into action is key to the growth and development of global health promotion [12]. Competencies provide a useful base for health promotion training and academic preparation, and guide the development of professional standards and systems of quality assurance in the field [12].

The literature on health promotion and health education competencies is repleted with frameworks and how they are developed. Discussion of the contexts influencing competency development, the value of the competency approach and the relationship between competencies and health promotion professionalization is also encountered [13]. The use of competencies for educational and practice settings is however less well defined when applied to HPS, particularly in resource–limited settings, and more research is needed to advance this field.

It is against this backdrop, that this chapter outlines the development of two HPS programs in South Africa, guided by work from doctoral research and a round table discussion on core health promotion competencies. The chapter focuses on: (a) the development, implementation, and evaluation of a HPS training program for high school educators in the Limpopo Province, guided by assessment of priority needs; and (b) factors influencing HPS implementation in three secondary schools in Cape Town. Attention is paid to training program objectives, learning outcomes, and critical cross-field outcomes related to introducing the HPS concept, empowerment of educators to initiate HPS and evaluate program design and implementation, and the key role of external actors and school stakeholders in designing and implementing HPS in these settings.

2. Health promoting schools (HPS) in South Africa

2.1 Development, implementation, and evaluation of a HPS training program for educators in Mankweng education circuit, Limpopo province

The first case study describes the capacity building of educators to enable HPS in Limpopo. The province is the northernmost part of South Africa and a typical developing region with a big gap between poor and rich residents, especially in rural areas. The population consists of several ethnic groups distinguished by culture, language, and race (97.3% black) and traditional leaders and chiefs still form a strong backbone of the political landscape. The study was conducted in the Mankweng area, a township adjacent to the University of Limpopo (pop 33,738) with eleven public high schools which fall under the control of the Department of Basic Education.

The study was informed by a needs assessment to inform the development of the HPS training program and guided by an eco-holistic framework for developing data collection instruments and the constructs of health promotion practice applicability in South African schools. The framework consisted of four external and five internal constructs that are interlinked in a dynamic interaction, highlighting the existence of, and interrelationship between factors at local, regional, national, and global level that influence HPS structure and development. The findings can guide future researchers in exploring skills among program planners and policy makers and how these skills influence health promotion practice in rural communities [14].

2.1.1 Needs assessment

The needs assessment used a sequential explanatory design with mixed method research, including a survey questionnaire for quantitative data collection among a representative sample of grade 9–11 learners (n=828) from eight randomly selected public schools in the area; semi-structured interviews with four key informants and in-depth interviews with seven student representatives. Ethics approval was granted by the Turfloop Research Ethics Committee and permission to conduct the study in the schools granted by the Department of Basic Education and other stakeholders. Informed consent was obtained in writing from the participants as well as parents of learners under the age of 18 years. Anonymity and confidentiality were guaranteed throughout the study.

The questionnaire included sections related to demographic and socioeconomic indicators, risk behavior, physical school environment and school climate and ethos. The questionnaire had been used in previous research in the area where its internal consistency had been established [15]; translated in the local language (Sepedi); and, administered by a trained researcher. The interview topic guide was grounded in the quantitative results. Instruments were pilot-tested before data collection and analysis was done descriptively for quantitative data and using Tesch's open coding technique for qualitative data analysis [16].

The most common *health risks* reported by learners included: (a) Substance use, particularly alcohol, followed by (b) sexual and reproductive health; and (c) bullying. Other substances apart from alcohol, included cigarettes and dagga smoking. Keeping more than one sexual partner was common and teenage pregnancy was frequently observed, even among learners in lower grades such as Grade 9, in line with previous studies [17, 18]. Unsafe sexual behaviour tends to be aggravated in rural and under-equipped schools as in Mankweng and other parts of Limpopo Province [19]. Many schools in rural areas also lack facilities such as dedicated sports grounds, and safety on the way to and from school is a health risk, especially for female learners vulnerable to crime.

Factors related to the *school climate* revealed the availability of safe clean water and garbage disposal in most schools, sufficient sanitation, discussion of health topics in the curriculum and learner involvement in local events. As regards *environmental and physical factors*, low cleanliness was reported in all schools, as well as vandalism, which is rampant and associated with gangsterism, school drop-outs, and ex-learners. Research indicate that juridical, economic, drugs and alcohol, and learner-related problems are important causes of vandalism [20]. Other environmental problems included cleanliness of toilets, safety and security, and the wider social environment.

Internal and external factors at school included issues related to management and planning, e.g., presence of a governing body and representative council of learners at each school. Ongoing evaluation of HPS highlighted several benefits that are part of school management objectives, including better learning outcomes, promoting staff health, creating a coordinated approach to social, physical as well as environmental needs. This study reported a need for HPS training of educators, in line with results from a study in the Western Cape [21], to enable learners to accept HPS. This was also linked to delays in the roll-out of the Life Skills program due to limited resources and capacity, especially in rural provinces such as the Eastern Cape and Limpopo.

Existing policies within the school environment provide for a course of action to address the social challenges faced by learners. Examples are the revised Integrated School Health Policy (2012) with a health education component on substance abuse.

The policy was developed to support learners to adopt health-promoting behaviors, but very little change has been observed, questioning the actual implementation of programs for optimal health. Educators only received training on programs such as Life Skills and HIV & AIDS Education, which is primarily located in the Life Orientation (LO) learning area/subject [22].

District office staff cannot visit and support schools often and effectively enough to ensure good quality education. Lack of skills, monitoring and accountability lead to poor policy implementation, inferior training of teachers and bureaucrats. Once-off interventions implemented by different service providers, including the Department of Health, Social Development, Education, and non-governmental organizations, is an approach that fails to bring behavior change among learners, and the LO curriculum does not take into account implementation of HPS, which requires skills that the LO educators do not possess [23].

The LO curriculum emphasizes the importance of skills, values and attitudes, and participation in physical activities and community initiatives, which are all elements of HPS [23]. Skills development of educators is therefore crucial to identify needs and implement continuous school-based programs such as the HPS initiative prescribed by WHO [24] to address health risk behavior that derail learners from achieving their educational goals. Selecting a priority issue can be used as a meaningful point of entry to guide HPS program development, using a sequence of well-defined steps outlined in the next section.

2.1.2 HPS training program development

A training program was developed to train educators in HPS in the study setting, based on a needs assessment, and comprising two-sessions that could be offered as a one to five days' workshop to ensure that relevant learning was addressed depending on the availability of educators. The first session introduced the HPS concept, and the training program goals, aligned to the WHO Information Series on School health, local action: Creating a Health Promoting School [24]. The second session covered the five steps of initiating HPS, using principles of adult learning guided by Knowles' theory of pedagogy and andragogy [25]. Next, guidelines for implementation of the training program were developed, followed by its implementation and evaluation.

The training program was designed to provide educators with a practical guide to HPS implementation and to achieve HPS accreditation in the Mankweng area using a series of five steps (**Box 1**).

Training program objectives, learning outcomes and critical cross-field outcomes focused on: introduction of the HPS concept and its benefits to educators; discussion of the association between health and education within school settings and the need for HPS; selecting priority problems as entry points to HPS training; introducing the steps to be followed when implementing HPS; and evaluating the training program. Learning outcomes were based on these objectives and described accordingly.

Although this was not a formal training program with any National Qualifications Framework level, as expected by the South African Qualifications Authority (SAQA) [27], critical cross-field outcomes (CCFOs) were considered important to guide the lifelong HPS related learning of educators. CCFOs are generic outcomes that inform teaching and learning, and they are deemed critical for building capacity for life-long learning. CCFOs related to this HPS training program were integrated in the material and methodology of the facilitator, and emphasized promotion of active, exploratory, and self-directed learning among educators [26].

Step 1: Understand what HPS is; solicit and achieve administrative and senior management buy-in and support; understand that HPS is a whole-school approach which needs ongoing support and commitment from school leaders.

Step 2: Create a task team to lead and coordinate health promotion activities. Key stakeholders should be represented on this group, including teachers, non-teaching staff, students, parents, and community members. The task team must share the workload, be involved in decision making and implementation, and conduct an audit of current needs and health promoting actions in line with the six components of the HPS framework [26].

Step 3: Establish agreed upon goals, objectives, and activities; develop strategies to achieve the goals with the available resources; develop a HPS Charter to symbolize the commitment of the school, setting out the school's principles and targets, and enabling the school to celebrate its achievements in health promotion. Staff should have opportunities to attend professional development programs and present and discuss their school initiatives with others.

Step 4: Take action, develop plans, and allocate tasks to different individuals according to their experiences and background. Engaging the community by identifying some individuals who have the skills to support HPS; create a supportive environment for HPS to flourish and support inter-sectoral collaboration.

Step 5: Monitoring and evaluation of all processes determining whether the goals and objectives for the identified priority areas are met. Methods must be identified to assess if planned activities and their implementation have been materialized. The school can be launched as HPS to showcase continuous strengthening of capacity to make schools a healthy setting to work, learn and live. Continuously assess if the five steps of HPS implementation are followed.

Box 1.
HPS training program implementation.

Educators should, for example, be able to: identify problems; formulate responses that demonstrate responsible decision-making where critical, and creative thinking; consider different ways of collecting and analyzing data, and evaluating information; work effectively in team, organization and the community; apply scientific skills and show accountability for creating a healthy school environment and looking after the health of others; and understand their environment as a set of interrelated systems by recognizing that problem-solving contexts do not exist in isolation [26].

Development of the HPS training program was informed by the WHO Information Series on HPS [24] and guided by Knowles' theory [25] around adult learning, which is based on the principles outlined below and adapted to the program (**Box 2**) [26].

2.1.3 HPS training program implementation and evaluation

The training with educators included data collection which reflected the current situation at participating schools. The focus was directed at risks the learners faced. HPS appeared to be a new concept to participants, and both learners and educators confirmed there were no programs and activities at their school focusing on learner health risk behavior, except for the nutrition program and physical activities, which were done occasionally in some schools outside examination time, and where social workers were deployed at school.

Program activities were based on the principles of adult learning outlined above and included assessment of participants' expectation of the training program as well as alignment with HPS training program content; explanation of the program topics and its relevance to HPS; sharing of experiences; ranking of health risk behaviors in the respective school settings; and a round of discussion to clarify areas of concern. These activities allowed participants to freely express themselves and engage in the

- Adult learners have a well-established sense of self which differs from previous life stages. It is equally important that educators as adults have their say in the training and autonomy in what they learn to keep their interest.
- Adults have past experiences, and the training program needs to feed into what they already know to be effective. Sharing of these experiences has to form part of the learning.
- As adults, educators, are purpose driven and motivated to learn when they see the relevance of the taught material. Hence only those who are willing to learn should attend the training as theory indicates that they will learn well.
- Internal motivation drives adults to develop their own ways of learning based on problem solving. Adults should not be expected to recite content but rather apply content in practice.
- During training, mistakes often become a valuable teacher. Learning happens when adults are allowed to explore the subject and learn from their mistakes.
- Adults need to play an active role in helping to design the course, personalize learning paths and select activities that are relevant to them and their work.

Box 2.
HPS training program principles.

HPS training program using Knowles' principles of adult learning, including building internal motivation, and capitalizing on individual experiences.

Participants rated the training program as good to excellent, indicating that the training program was an eye opener to responsibilities, which they were not aware of [26]. Participants did not know that there were formal initiatives which could assist schools, parents, learners, and educators to address challenges hampering teaching and learning at school and enhance school health [26]. Educators agreed that their expectations had been met and the imparted knowledge would improve their ability to perform their jobs. They indicated that the training was well planned, informative, empowering, technical, and relevant for application in their school contexts.

2.2 Factors influencing HPS implementation: a multiple case study of three secondary schools in a resource-limited community in Cape Town

2.2.1 Introduction

In the Western Cape, an HPS project was conducted driven by the need to reduce the spread of TB and HIV in secondary schools. The project was funded by the Centers for Disease Control and Prevention and conducted over a period of three and a half years in a resource-limited area with high rates of TB and HIV close to the University of the Western Cape (UWC). The project team comprised an educational psychologist; two members from the Faculty of Education; two from Physiotherapy & Occupational Therapy; one from the School of Public Health; and a school doctor employed by the Provincial Department of Health. This diverse range of expertise and experience was an advantage as it drew on different paradigms because of the different backgrounds.

After an initial workshop to introduce the HPS concept and approach, a series of workshops was held in each school at the start of the project with teachers, students, and parents, as well as a workshop with all schools together [28]. The aim of the first workshop was to identify the needs in the school community around health and well-being, while the second workshop focused on TB and HIV [28]. In groups, participants brainstormed what was already in place to address the challenges of TB and HIV. Using the information from the two workshops, each school subsequently drew up its own plan of action, bearing in mind what was realistically achievable.

Although the funding aimed at capacity development for TB and HIV prevention, the project team used this as an entry point for HPS implementation. The focus was on generic capacity building across the schools. Once the participants became familiar with the HPS approach and the social determinants of TB and HIV, they developed their own agendas based on their perceived relevance and priority [28]. The value of these workshops was that teachers, students, and parents (to a lesser extent) worked together towards realizing the goal of HPS project implementation because they were receptive to its benefits.

2.2.2 Project process and approach

The project team subscribed to certain processes and approaches to facilitate HPS implementation. A HPS committee was formed at each school comprising of teachers, students, and parents (to some extent). A member of the UWC team was appointed to each school to guide implementation via monthly meetings with the HPS committee and separate *ad hoc* meetings with students and teachers. The team was also directly involved in HPS planning in the initial stages but took a more facilitative role later on.

A participatory approach was used based on the Appreciative Inquiry technique, which applies a positive stance and builds on organizational strengths to encourage growth and development [29]. For example, the HPS committees were asked to draw a dream tree depicting their ambition and a mapping exercise to outline the available resources. The teams worked with those who were receptive and eager to be involved and remained flexible in allowing schools to advance at their own pace and focus on their own plans.

A student camp was held each year focusing on leadership and empowerment to build capacity among students to implement HPS and develop as an individual. The value of the camp was that students were encouraged to explore and reflect on their feelings and capabilities independently of teachers or parents—an opportunity they did not often have. The camp was facilitated by members of the UWC team in addition to other organizations with expertise in youth development, communications, team building and TB and HIV.

2.2.3 Role of the external partner

Studies report that schools often lack the skills and competence to implement any health-promoting change, and hence need external catalysts for change [30, 31]. In this project, the UWC team was perceived as crucial for facilitating implementation. Apart from some financial and material support, they provided technical assistance, e.g., through workshops and skills development activities. Some teachers attended a short course at UWC to improve their HPS skills. The team also provided mentorship, guidance, education, and problem solving with the local HPS school committee.

The team was also seen as giving direction while receiving first-hand information of what was happening in the external and internal social context of the school. The nature of the collaboration of the UWC team with the school was in keeping with the settings approach of using a participatory bottom-up approach right from the start of the project, and its role was perceived as resulting in a valuable relationship with the school: "*... without your involvement... and input I don't think this school would have opened many other doors...*" (Teacher, AP3).

Relationship building was also a key role of the school facilitator, who confirmed that through constant in-person interaction a good relationship had been established with the HPS group and the school in general. The facilitator claimed that this contact provided an opportunity to feel the rhythm of the school, enabling to fit in with the way the school functioned. The facilitator felt that this was necessary to consolidate HPS and keep it on the school agenda, a finding which is consistent with other studies on the guiding and supporting role of school health advisors [30].

The findings of this study indicate that as initiators of the HPS concept, one of the key roles of the UWC team was to ascertain that the HPS concept was understood as a *whole-school* approach and implemented in a way that suited the schools. Its role was hence facilitative and enabling rather than effecting HPS implementation, in line with the findings of Boot et al. [30], which showed that practical assistance, building a trusting relationship and showing proof of professional skills and knowledge were important mechanisms for school advisors to facilitate project implementation.

The team acknowledged that the school knew what was best for them and were "experts" in terms of their own contexts. The team saw reciprocal learning as being crucial to a shared understanding of HPS and its requirements, which was especially important in view of applying a settings approach. The team worked with different actors in the school system (principal, teachers, parents, and students) which allowed them to gain a better understanding of the context and degrees of commitment of the actors and to gain their trust, which is a key aspect of collaborative work [32].

In keeping with the settings approach, the team further networked with external organizations and institutions that could provide services and resources that were conducive to HPS implementation. Implementation of the HPS program was however influenced by internal and contextual factors, which compromised how it was able to effectively implement the integration of HPS as a whole-school approach, all of which could have an impact on whether HPS was to be sustainable in this context [28].

2.2.4 Building capacity for HPS implementation

In this project, capacity building of students was key to facilitate participation in HPS project implementation. Capacity building resulted not only in personal benefits but also contributed to a positive implementation climate by creating an empowering environment. Students from the participating schools attended the leadership camps where skills were developed to implement HPS. In two schools, students were able to put these leadership and other skills to use by taking some responsibility and fulfilling certain roles for HPS.

Although it was clear from this project that students across participating schools had gained knowledge and an understanding of health in its holistic sense, and were committed to the implementation of HPS, findings also indicated that student action differed from school to school. The levels of competence and involvement varied and were influenced by school climate and culture, the internal support received from the headmaster and other staff members, peers, the principal, and the external support received from the UWC team and other external agents.

Student empowerment indeed carries an understanding that, while students have a sense of agency, they need support and guidance from their teachers to support the implementation climate. In this study, students worked closely with the teachers they trusted, who respected and accepted them as persons and who listened to their ideas. This demonstrates the powerful role teachers can play in providing opportunities for students to realize their potential, which happens rarely because of the community context and school culture of excluding students from decision-making [33].

It was evident from the study that, where the students had specific, clearly defined roles in the HPS project, they had a sense of purpose and felt valued since they were trying to make a meaningful difference [28]. Being seen as resources or assets rather than cases increases the chance of empowerment among young people as they will be seen as having the skills and knowledge to bring about change for themselves [32]. Where students are perceived as unequal partners, they may feel disempowered and consequently could become disengaged from HPS [34].

The benefits of HPS involvement for teachers were not evident in this study. This could be because teacher involvement carried more responsibilities than for students or other staff. The benefits for teachers hence cannot be perceived to be similar as for students who only seemed to gain from their involvement, while for some teachers it may have added to their workload. It has been recommended that capacity building for teachers should indeed not only aim at implementing HPS, but also at encouraging and gaining support from and working in partnership with, their peers and other actors [35].

Although some efforts were done by school facilitators to facilitate partnerships through mentoring and guiding of students and teachers, other contextual factors negatively influenced the ability to fully implement HPS as a whole- school approach, including a strike by teachers, and work and personal commitments. One attempt at building capacity among staff was when the UWC team shared the results of their HPS school climate survey with individual schools, giving staff an opportunity to engage and assess how they could integrate it into the curriculum and other school functions.

At the workshop, participants seemed to fully engage with the information, and teachers discussed how they could use it across the curriculum. The UWC team made further attempts to build the capacities of the teachers and staff directly involved in HPS, including organizing a camp to develop understanding of the HPS concept and process and facilitating a short course on HPS, which was attended by some teachers [28]. The activities took place during school holidays, which also meant that teachers had to compromise on their free time to be able to attend the training.

The fact they did this willingly reflects their readiness for change and commitment to building HPS capacity. On the other hand, teachers were not given an opportunity to further build their capacity or put into practice their acquired skills as part of the normal school operations. This might have resulted in teachers feeling less valued for their work and hence not taking ownership of the program [28]. If HPS would have been implemented as a whole-school approach, time would have been allocated to build capacity for HPS implementation by leadership and management.

A key finding related to capacity building was the challenge of continuity due to staff turnover. This had repercussions in terms of the quality of implementation and sustainability, especially if the leaving staff member carried a high responsibility for HPS implementation. This again could have been averted if a whole-school approach had been taken. Where responsibilities were shared, the potential for integration in the school life was greater. Therefore, leadership capacity must be built at different levels to complement, and, if required, succeed those in leadership positions.

3. Discussion

In the last decades, HPS has become widely accepted as the gold standard for implementing health promotion in school environments, and evidence has indicated its effectiveness [36]. In South Africa, the concept has gained traction since the advent of democracy and the two case studies described in this chapter are testimony to that. The case studies describe attempts to implement HPS in disadvantaged communities based on its value system by imparting knowledge and understanding of the concept; building capacity in terms of leadership and management skills; and communication with, and empowerment of students and educators.

Taken together, these competencies are in line with the set of core competencies for health promotion as outlined in existing competency frameworks, e.g., the Galway Consensus Statement for Health Promotion Competencies [37]. The core domains of competency agreed to in the Consensus Statement are catalyzing change, leadership, assessment, planning, implementation, evaluation, advocacy, and partnerships, all of which were adhered to a greater or lesser extent in the case studies described above. In Limpopo, educators were trained through a rigorous process of induction into HPS concept and methodology, showing proof of acquired competencies in terms of HPS knowledge and understanding. In Cape Town, the focus was on capacity building, and HPS implementation highlighted the key role of students as agents of change.

In the latter study, students showcased their role based on their newly acquired competencies of leadership and project management skills. Constant communication of school-based facilitators with the local HPS committee was also found to facilitate HPS implementation and enabled continuous buy-in and sustained implementation. In addition, results indicate that the UWC team consciously tried to practice cultural humility by not setting the agenda [38], which minimizes the power balance between partners [39], including professionals and communities, by valuing lay knowledge [40] and cultivating mutual respect [41].

The value placed on communication and cultural humility were also found to be core health promotion competencies for South Africa as identified in a round table on core competencies for health promotion organized at UWC in 2014. The round table gathered stakeholders involved in health promotion from academia, government, and civil society and found that the existing core competency frameworks, with particular attention to the CompHP Core Competencies Framework for Health Promotion [42] were useful, but lacked some specific competencies for the region.

Participants at the round table also concluded that health promotion training in South Africa should match the need for specific skills and that service training should be developed next to academic curricula. Attention towards cultural competency and health literacy and knowledge management were considered equally important as the higher outlined core competency domains. To meet these expectations, strategic engagement between training institutions, government and civil society was deemed necessary to formulate the appropriate competencies.

In the above-described case studies, the aim was to build capacity in terms of HPS implementation; and to instill confidence and competencies to implement and sustain HPS even after support of the external facilitators ceased. Studies suggest that teacher training and professional development are required to enable them to act as catalysts for change [43–46]. Similarly, capacity building of students was found to be crucial for HPS implementation in the second case study. The findings indeed show that capacity building of students resulted not only in personal gains, but contributed to a positive HPS implementation climate [47].

Many studies report that schools do not have the skills and competence to achieve health-promoting changes, and hence need external catalysts for change [30, 31]. For example, universities have been found to play an important role as external catalysts by creating a supportive climate for HPS implementation in schools [41, 48, 49].The first case study shows that the development, implementation and evaluation of a HPS Training Program provides evidence that skills development of school educators improves HPS knowledge and understanding and creates an enabling environment where students learn how to control health risks and practice health behaviour [26].

The HPS program also assisted learners to achieve educational outcomes and enhance the health and well-being of all those involved [26]. The Training Program improved knowledge, understanding and skills around HPS, and addressed health risks, physical and environmental challenges, the school climate, and ethos issues of implementing a whole-of-school approach.

The second study also revealed how the program assisted actors at different levels of the school system to identify the link between what they were already doing and the HPS approach [28]. Where a link to existing practice and processes was in place, it was easier to integrate new initiatives such as HPS [46]. Seeing these links increased the readiness for change, although this understanding was not enough for the schools to achieve full integration of HPS. One of the values implicit in the settings approach was also participation of those affected or targeted for health promotion initiatives, including teachers and students, as described in the two case studies.

The UWC team acted as an external catalyst, ensuring that the HPS concept was understood as a whole-school approach and implemented in the best way that suited the school and implementers. The team saw its role as facilitative and enabling, rather than effecting HPS implementation. The team used reciprocal learning to achieve a shared understanding of what HPS entails, which was especially appropriate in terms of the settings approach, in which different stakeholders (principal, teachers, parents and students) were invited to gain more understanding of the context and degrees of commitment of these actors. This also allowed to gain their trust, which is important in collaborative working [32]. With this knowledge, the team was able to ascertain what the schools' concerns were and what was needed, and through HPS strategies attempted to respond to some of these issues in partnership with the different actors [41, 50], consistent with the settings approach and the practice of cultural humility.

Although teachers in the second case study attempted to empower students and implement HPS, they lacked the skills to do so. They were not supported by the school or education authorities to develop these skills [28]. Even teachers who attended the short course were not supported, indicating that HPS is not a high-ranking priority and showcasing the barriers teachers and students face when trying to implement HPS. Hence the question of how realistic any HPS approach can be, considering the diverse needs and heterogeneity within a particular school, comes to mind. This could also be the reason why some teachers and students did not become involved in HPS.

In the South Africa education sector, health issues are addressed mainly as part of the life skills curriculum with little room and time for active student participation and critical reflection. A top-down approach to education is typically used, which does not allow much space for teachers and students to experiment with HPS. There seems to be a lack of political will from the education and health sectors to work collaboratively towards the health and well-being of young people, which highlight the difficulty of implementing HPS as a whole school approach, raising the question of whether it is idealistic to achieve HPS in a context such as of the above-described case studies.

The implication for HPS in South Africa is that, unless there is sufficient political will to create an environment in which a whole school HPS approach can be realized and its value and potential appreciated by all stakeholders, it will be an uphill battle for those wanting to implement HPS. Using incremental changes can be an effective lever to achieve organizational readiness for change, starting with marginal changes in activities and the commitment of those involved [28]. Once the changes are visible schools could be tempted to attempt more complex changes. Hence striving towards implementation of HPS as a whole school approach is a goal worth pursuing for South African youth to be able to make a meaningful contribution to society.

4. Conclusion

This chapter described two case studies of HPS implementation in South Africa. The first case study showed how the implementation of a HPS training program for educators in the Mankweng Education Circuit, Limpopo Province, could be used for skills development of educators in addressing problems that typically interfere with teaching and learning. Recognizing that the entire school community is important, educators were encouraged to initiate HPS programs. Educators agreed that instead of inviting professionals for ad hoc support, they wanted to develop a sustainable program to empower learners to take care of their own health behavior.

The second case study highlighted the significant contribution that students can make in HPS implementation. Students were found to be key assets with the potential to take responsibility for many practices and processes of program implementation. Student participation and building leadership capacity should hence be a major aim of HPS implementation in secondary schools. If students are given enough autonomy, they can develop a sense of agency and ability, which is especially important in view of the heavy workload of teachers who usually carry the bulk of HPS implementation.

Taken together, the case studies illustrate the role of competency building among both educators and students to implement HPS programs in secondary schools that result in capacity and motivation to transform the educational environment in South Africa into an environment that enables educators and learners to achieve their full health potential.

Author details

Joyce Mashamba[1], Suraya Mohamed[2], Peter Delobelle[2,3,4]* and Hans Onya[5]

1 Department of Public Health, University of Limpopo, Mankweng, South Africa

2 School of Public Health, University of the Western Cape, Bellville, South Africa

3 Department of Medicine, University of Cape Town, Cape Town, South Africa

4 Department of Public Health, Vrije Universiteit Brussel, Brussels, Belgium

5 Research Development and Administration, University of Limpopo, Mankweng, South Africa

*Address all correspondence to: pdelobelle@gmail.com

References

[1] WHO. Ottawa Charter for Health Promotion. in International Conference on Health Promotion. Ottawa, Canada: s.n; 1986

[2] St. Leger L et al. In: McQueen DV, Jones CM, editors. School Health Promotion: Achievements, Challenges and Priorities, in Global Perspectives on Health Promotion Effectiveness. New York: Springer; 2007. pp. 107-124

[3] WHO. Health-Promoting Schools : A Healthy Setting for Living, Learning and Working. Geneva: World Health Organization; 1998

[4] WHO. WHO Guideline on School Health Services. Geneva: World Health Organization; 2021

[5] Swart D, Reddy P. Establishing Networks for Health Promoting Schools in South Africa. Journal of School Health. 1999;**69**(2):47

[6] Lazarus S. Executive Summary, National Health Promoting Schools Conference 14–16 September 2006. Cape Town, South Africa: University of the Western Cape; 2006

[7] Mukoma W, Flisher AJ. Evaluations of health promoting schools: A review of nine studies. Health Promotion International. 2004;**19**(3):357-368

[8] DOH. The National Health Promotion Policy and Strategy 2015–2019. Pretoria: Department of Health; 2015

[9] Shilton T et al. Health promotion development, and health promotion workforce competency in Australia: An historical overview. Health Promotion Journal of Australia: Official Journal of Australian Association of Health Promotion Professionals. 2001;**12**:117-123

[10] WHO and UNESCO. Making Every School a Health-Promoting School—Global Standards and Indicators. Geneva: World Health Organization and the United Nations Educational, Scientific and Cultural Organization; 2021

[11] WHO. Making Every School a Health-Promoting School—Country Case Studies. 2021. Available from: https://www.who.int/publications/i/item/9789240025431

[12] Battel-Kirk B et al. A review of the international literature on health promotion competencies: identifying frameworks and core competencies. Global Health Promotion. 2009;**16**(2):12-20

[13] WHO. Global School Health Initiatives: Achieving Health and Education Outcomes: Report of a Meeting, Bangkok, Thailand, 23–25 November 2015. Geneva: World Health Organization; 2017

[14] Taherdoost H. Validity and reliability of the research instrument; how to test the validation of a questionnaire/survey in research. International Journal of Academic Research in Management. 2016;**5**:28-36. DOI: 10.2139/ssrn.3205040

[15] Aaro LE et al. An HIV/AIDS knowledge scale for adolescents: item response theory analyses based on data from a study in South Africa and Tanzania. Health Education Research. 2011;**26**(2):212-224

[16] Creswell JW. Qualitative Inquiry and Research Design: Choosing Among Five Approaches. 3rd ed. Thousand Oaks: SAGE Publications; 2012

[17] Reddy S et al. Umthente Uhlaba Usamila—The South African Youth Risk

Behaviour Survey 2008. Cape Town: South African Medical Research Council; 2010

[18] Onya H et al. Adolescent alcohol use in rural South African high schools. African Journal of Psychiatry (Johannesbg). 2012;**15**(5):352-357

[19] Stats SA. Census 2011. Pretoria: Statistics South Africa; 2011

[20] De Wet C. The extent and causes of learner vandalism at schools. South African Journal of Education. 2004; **24**(3):206-211

[21] Waggie F, Laattoe N, Filies GC. Moving from conversation to commitment: Optimising school-based health promotion in the Western Cape, South Africa. African Journal of Health Professions Education. 2013; **5**(1):26-29

[22] Department of Basic Education. Health Promotion. 2021. Available from: https://www.education.gov.za/Programmes/HealthPromotion/tabid/672/Default.aspx [Accessed: January 16, 2021]

[23] Jacobs A. Life orientation as experienced by learners: A qualitative study in North-West Province. South African Journal of Education. 2011;**3**(2): 212-223

[24] WHO. Local Action: Creating Health-Promoting Schools. Geneva: World Health Organization; 2000

[25] Knowles MS. The Modern Practice of Adult Education: From Pedagogy to Andragogy. 2nd ed. New York: Cambridge University Press; 1980

[26] Mashamba T. Development, Implementation and Evaluation of a Health Promoting School Training Programme for Educators in High Schools of Mankweng Circuit, Limpopo Province, South Africa. Thesis submitted in Fulfilment of the Requirements for the Degree Doctor of Philosophy in Health Sciences. University of Limpopo; 2021

[27] SAQA. The South African Qualifications Authority: Level Descriptors for South African National Qualifications Framework. Waterkloof: South African Qualifications Authority; 2012

[28] Mohamed S. Factors influencing the implementation of health promoting schools: A multiple case study of three secondary schools in a resource limited community in Cape Town. Thesis submitted in fulfilment of the requirements for the degree Doctor in Philosophy in Health Sciences. University of the Western Cape; 2015

[29] Bryan KS, Klein DA, Elias MJ. Applying organizational theories to action research in community settings: A case study in Urban schools. Journal of Community Psychology. 2007;**35**(3): 383-398

[30] Boot N et al. Professional assistance in implementing school health policies. Health Education. 2010;**110**(4):294-308

[31] Bruce E, Klein R, Keleher H. Parliamentary inquiry into health promoting schools in Victoria: Analysis of stakeholder views. Journal of School Health. 2012;**82**(9):441-447

[32] Jones J, Barry MM. Exploring the relationship between synergy and partnership functioning factors in health promotion partnerships. Health Promotion International. 2011;**26**(4):408-420

[33] El Ansari CJPW. Partnerships, community participation and intersectoral collaboration in South Africa. Journal of Interprofessional Care. 2001;**15**(2):119-132

[34] Harrist CJ. Hearing voices. A response to "Case Study of a Participatory Health-Promotion Intervention in School". Democracy and Education [Internet]. 2011;**20**(1). Available from: https://democracyeducationjournal.org/home/vol20/iss1/10

[35] Bond L, Glover S, Godfrey C, Butler H, Patton GC. Building capacity for system-level change in schools: Lessons from the Gatehouse Project. Health Education & Behavior, 2001;**28**(3):368-383. Doi:10.1177/109019810102800310

[36] Wagner GH et al. Health promoting schools evidence for effectiveness—Action lab report. Promotion and Education. 2003;**10**(4):182-185

[37] Barry MM et al. The galway consensus conference: International collaboration on the development of core competencies for health promotion and health education. Global Health Promotion. 2009;**16**(2):5-11

[38] Tervalon M, Murray-Garcia J. Cultural humility versus cultural competence: a critical distinction in defining physician training outcomes in multicultural education. Journal of Health Care for the Poor and Underserved. 1998;**9**(2):117-125

[39] Milbourne L, Macrae S, Maguire M. Collaborative solutions or new policy problems: Exploring multi-agency partnerships in education and health work. Journal of Education Policy. 2003;**18**(1):19-35

[40] Minkler M. Community-based research partnerships: Challenges and opportunities. Journal of Urban Health. 2005;**82**(2 Suppl. 2):ii3-i12

[41] Butler J et al. Utilizing the school health index to build collaboration between a university and an urban school district. Journal of School Health. 2011;**81**(12):774-782

[42] Barry MM, Battel-Kirk B, Dempsey C. The CompHP core competencies framework for health promotion in Europe. Health Education & Behavior. 2012;**39**(6):648-662

[43] Aldinger C et al. Strategies for implementing Health-Promoting Schools in a province in China. Promotion and Education. 2008;**15**(1):24-29

[44] Hoyle TB, Bartee R, Allensworth DD. Applying the process of health promotion in schools: A commentary. The Journal of School Health. 2010;**80**(4):163-166

[45] Lochman JE. Commentary: School contextual influences on the dissemination of interventions. School Psychology Review. 2003;**32**(2):174-177

[46] Pommier J, Guevel MR, Jourdan D. A health promotion initiative in French primary schools based on teacher training and support: Actionable evidence in context. Global Health Promotion. 2011;**18**(1):34-38

[47] Cargo M et al. Empowerment as fostering positive youth development and citizenship. American Journal of Health Behavior. 2003;**27**(Suppl. 1):S66-S79

[48] Inchley J, Currie C, Young I. Evaluating the health promoting school: a case study approach. Health Education. 2000;**100**(5):200-206

[49] Preiser R et al. External stakeholders and health promoting schools: Complexity and practice in South Africa. Health Education. 2014;**114**(4):260-270

[50] Dumka LE, Mauricio A-M, Gonzales NA. Research partnerships with schools to implement prevention programs for Mexican origin families. The Journal of Primary Prevention. 2007;**28**(5):403-420

Chapter 6

Physical Education Teacher's Professional Learning of Implementing a Health Promotion Intervention in the Practice of a Research Circle

Linn Håman, Katarina Haraldsson and Eva-Carin Lindgren

Abstract

Scholars recommend that health promotion researchers engage practitioners in the analysis and reporting phase and expand their ability to share their research beyond academia. The purpose of this study was to draw benefit from physical education (PE) teachers' discussions and reflections of the implementation of a health promotion intervention in school during research circle meetings. The health promotion intervention 'Pulse for Health and Learning' (PuLH) focused on moderate-to-vigorous physical activity, incorporating a child-centred coaching approach. This study has an action research approach. The research circle consisted of PE teachers (N = 22, approximately 18 per meeting) from eight primary and middle schools (from grades 4 to 9) in eight municipalities in Sweden and three researchers. The theory of 'practice architectures' was employed to interpret, discuss, and clarify what enables and constrain PE teachers' implementation of the health promotion intervention. During the analysis, three discourses were identified: technical-rational discourse, participating discourse, and steering and supporting discourse. The practice architectures both enabled and constrained the implementation of PuLH. The research circle meetings stimulated critically conscious acting and decision-making through collaboration between PE teachers and together with researchers which improved the implementation of PuLH and contributed to PE teachers' professional development.

Keywords: action research approach, health promotion, implementation, intervention, moderate-to-vigorous physical activity, physical education, professional development, research circle, school

1. Introduction

Schools are considered essential for health promotion interventions [1], but several complex aspects are necessary for successful implementation [2–4]—for instance, teamwork, leadership, assistance, and contextual factors [2, 3]. Likewise, the competence of the individual teachers and support from the organization they work within is necessary [5]. Through practice-developing school research, teachers' professional knowledge base can be strengthened and developed [6]. Continuing professional learning among teachers is necessary for supporting and encouraging the improvement of knowledge and practice (e.g., [7]). One way to keep this is by conducting different forms of professional development programs for teachers in school (e.g., [7]). Previous research has shown that professional development positively influences teachers' capacity to reflect on new knowledge and practices [8]. It could be significant to teacher professional learning [9]. Teachers will suffer from a lack of professional learning if they are alone for most of their working time, do not receive feedback and support from their colleagues, and do not have contact with teachers at other schools [10]. Collaborative reflection [11] and 'shared values and vision, collegiality and joint practical activities' have been identified as essential parts of professional learning programs [12]. Moreover, scholars describe that professional learning is based on research, engagement, and agency and that teachers are considered active producers instead of recipients of knowledge (e.g., [7, 13]). However, professional communities for learning need architecture or a design; if they are to produce results, they must be organized and arranged [10].

One way of working with professional communities for learning or collegial learning in schools is through so-called research circles, in which teachers and researchers collaborate on specific content [7, 14–16]. Research circles can be regarded as an action research approach, where researchers and practitioners see the process as a collective work [17]. Thus, the action research approach means, for instance, that those affected by the study are involved in joint exploratory work throughout the process on equal terms [17]. A previous study that has used research circles showed that the collaboration and reflections contributed to improvements in their daily professional practices [7]. Furthermore, the teachers anchored their experiences from the research circle in their preschool development plans [7]. Another study among teachers in schools showed that the research circle worked to deepen the development of teachers' competencies [16]. A conclusion from a recent study with teachers who had participated in research circles stresses the importance of when researchers and practitioners work together to translate research-based knowledge and theoretical concepts into practice and specify how practitioners can apply it when developing their actions [18].

Moreover, a study about school leader perspectives shows that they perceived it as an advantage that the teachers who participated in a research circle could exchange experiences from their everyday practice. Another benefit from the school leaders' perspective was that the researchers were necessary for the processes generated in the research circle. For example, they acted as catalysts for the conversation and the ideas that arose [15]. However, there are also challenges surrounding the implementation of a research circle and for example, not having suitable organizational conditions and getting enough time and space aside for the work. Despite this, it can be difficult for teachers to have enough time to participate. Another challenge may be that many teachers at the school are not included in the development work if the research circle focuses on a limited number of teachers, e.g., physical education (PE) teachers [15]. Research circles build on work that fits well in schools since education must be based on scientific grounds and proven experience [19]. In this context, practice-based research projects have a role to fill [6, 20] since teachers can continue professional learning based on research. This is important from a health promotion perspective where participation and capacity building are highlighted [5, 21]. Moreover, scholars [22] recommend that health-promoting researchers engage users in the analysis and reporting phase and expand their ability to share their research outside academia.

In this study, physical education (PE) teachers collaborated with the researchers (the study's authors) in a research circle consisting of three meeting practices. The ambition was to increase professional learning regarding developing and implementing a health-promoting intervention (the Pulse for Health and Learning Intervention, PuLH) which incorporated a child-centred coaching approach. PuLH lasted for one academic year and focused on three mandated moderate-to-vigorous physical activity (MVPA) sessions per week which lasted 30 min. The pupils were supposed to be in a heart rate zone between 60% and 80% of their maximum heart rate for at least 20 min. The MVPA sessions were implemented for pupils in primary and middle school, in addition to the two ordinary PE lessons [23]. The purpose of this study was to draw benefit from physical education teachers' discussions and reflections of the implementation of PuLH, a health promotion intervention in school. The questions to be addressed are; (1) How do the practice architectures enable and constrain the PE teachers' implementation of PuLH? and (2) What discourses are visible in the PE teachers' discussions and reflections of the implementation of PuLH?.

2. Theoretical framework

The development of professional learning among individual health promoters is a necessity but not a sufficient prerequisite for achieving effective health promotion work. The staff in an organization also need, for example, the support of their principals and colleagues and the resources needed to effectively implement health-promoting strategies [5]. The theory of 'practice architectures' [24] is used in this study to interpret, discuss and make sense of what PE teachers' discussed during the research circle about the implementation. Namely, what discourses had enabled and constrained their implementation of PuLH. The theory comprises three interrelated dimensions: cultural-discursive, material-economic, and socio-political arrangements [25]. The arrangements in the theory of practice architectures are structures that influence what is possible to say, do, and how one relates to each other in specific situations that influence practice. The arrangements can, just like the practice, be analytically distinguished, but they are also interwoven. These arrangements form the architectures of practice that enable and constrain or even hinder it [24].

Cultural-discursive arrangements are influenced by what is possible to say and talk about in a specific context and place in a particular time. The PE teachers' speeches in practice are influenced by how they talk about PuLH, what they can do, what is possible to do both in the local context and by discourses that exist both nationally and internationally. The PE teachers' speeches might also shape the tradition of sharing knowledge and reflecting on developing new ways of talking about content in PuLH, form, conditions for implementation, etc. Thus, the arrangements might shape the PE teachers' speeches about content and new ways of 'doing' to understand the role as an implementer and the knowledge that is important for creating new strategies and solutions for developing PuLH.

Material-economic arrangements influence opportunities for collaboration and meetings in practice. The research circle might enable PE teachers to collaborate and reflect on the implementation of PuLH. But, the time and place for meetings in the research circle influence the opportunity for everyone to meet. Material-economic arrangements also influence the opportunities that exist in the PE teachers' practice to, for example, be able to conduct the PuLH sessions with suitable facilities and equipment.

Socio-political arrangements influence how PE teachers relate to each other. For example, how the PE teachers share their experiences of running PuLH, what activities they do, how the activities work, how they support each other in the development work. These arrangements shape practice based on power, communication, and approaches. Since a research circle is based on participation and collaboration, PE teachers have the opportunity to contribute with knowledge to each other. In addition, the schools' different decisions about PuLH condition the PE teachers' opportunities to run PuLH.

The arrangements keep practices in place, and for a practice to change, the arrangements must also change. In turn, a practice can also contribute to changing the arrangements and influence other practices (a local practice can also influence an entire municipality) [25]. Therefore, it is not only the specific practice that is studied but also its arrangement.

3. Method

This study has an action research approach [26] using research circles that aim to understand and change PE teachers' practices and the conditions that enable and constrain them. The action research approach requires PE teachers to inquire into their practices and is, by nature, participatory [27]. This implies that action research in this study aims to promote change derived from and responsive to the PE teachers' commonly addressed ideas and concerns, grounded firmly in their experiences.

3.1 Setting

The Pulse for Health and Learning Intervention (PuLH) was conducted in eight mixed socio-economic municipalities (population 7000–30,000 inhabitants) in the region of Jönköping, Sweden. The PuLH-intervention involved eight primary and middle schools from grades 4 to 9 (see reference [23] for a more detailed description of the PuLH intervention). During the PuLH-intervention, PE teachers in charge at each school participated in a collegial learning research circle (cf. [28]).

3.2 Research circle

PuLH was a practice-based health promotion intervention, and the initiative to start the PuLH intervention arose from schools' need to increase pupils' chances of improving their grades [23]. The idea of the intervention was based on some research showing that physical activity (PA) and MVPA correlated with pupils' academic performance [29–31] and that MVPA has a beneficial effect on their health [32, 33]. In this study, the research circle consisted of three full days of research circle meetings: in September 2017, in December 2017, and May 2018. The researchers, PE teachers, and each municipality's development managers planned to conduct the research circle. The research circle process was an iterative process where PE teachers discuss

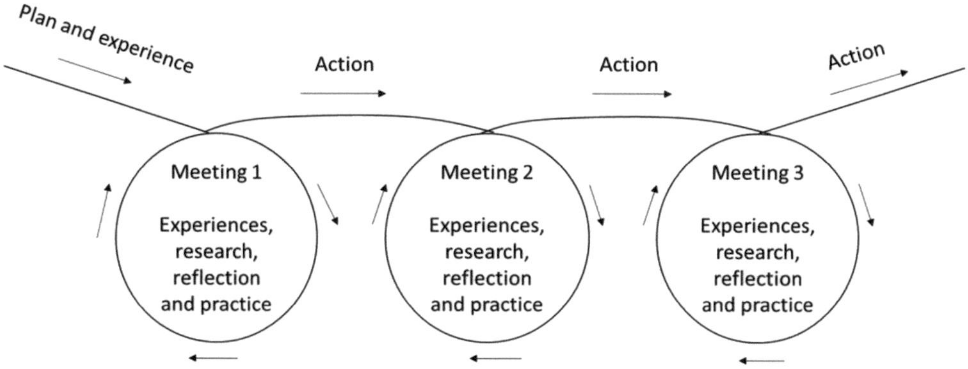

Figure 1.
The research circle process.

dilemmas and the content in the meetings with researchers, plan for a new act, and then act and so on (**Figure 1**).

The research circle was arranged to reflect in discussions the experiences of the implementation of PuLH and increase PE teachers' understanding of a coaching approach to include all children. The PE teacher's knowledge of their practice in the PuLH was also in focus, and discussions and reading aimed to give new insights to improve practice. The goal was to provide the PE teachers with conditions that enable them to change their practice and address the constraints satisfactorily (i.e., [34, 35]). Indeed, previous research has shown the value of researchers and practitioners working together [18, 22].

Activities were undertaken on a shared electronic platform between the three research circle meetings. This virtual space was supportive and allowed everybody to prepare and express their ideas and views for the meetings and read texts and scientific articles distributed by the researchers. During the research circle meetings, the researchers contributed to the process of relating the PE teachers' knowledge about their practices to scientific knowledge in a critical way.

We divided the PE teachers into two groups (A and B). At each meeting, the groups were mixed to receive input from different PE teachers and schools. Group A started to participate in lectures and applied workshops, and group B discussed experiences of the implementation of PuLH. After that, the groups switched. The researcher in charge at Halmstad University led each research circle meeting, and the two other researchers were observers. The first research circle meeting focused on health promotion and a child-centred coaching approach. The second meeting covered self-determination theory (SDT) concerning coaching. The third meeting focused on MVPA activities for pupils with disabilities and a presentation of preliminary results on the pupils' voices of PuLH [23] which we jointly reflected and discussed. The researcher asked relevant questions in the discussions but had a lowkey during the discussions. During the discussions, the PE teachers were encouraged to exchange experiences of the implementation of PuLH. Researchers led the lecture, and PE teacher educators led the applied workshops.

The first two research circle meetings were held at the conference room distributed by the Department of Research and Development within Education, Region Jönköping County, and the last one at Halmstad University.

3.3 Participants

The participants were PE teachers (N = 22, approximately 18 per meeting) from eight different primary and middle schools. The PE teachers represented a wide span, from a few years to those with several years of experience in the profession. At the beginning of the research circle meetings, only a few PE teachers had the experience of running MVPA activities at schools.

3.4 Data collection and ethical considerations

The data consist of group discussions, (n = 6) audio-recorded and transcribed verbatim in the research circle meetings. The transcribed empirical data amounted to 302 pages, Times new roman 12 points, double line spacing.

The PE teachers permitted to participate in the study and were informed of its purpose. They were ensured the data could not be traced to individual respondents or workplaces. The principles concern that all participants provided written consent and confidentiality. The Regional Ethics Review Board of Lund University approved this study (DNR 217/601), and the research follows The Swedish Research Council's guidelines [36].

3.5 Data analysis

The first and last author conducted the data analysis. However, to reach a consensus in the data analysis, all research group members discussed all phases and steps. An abductive data analysis approach was adopted [37], which allowed us to engage in a dialectic process of considering data and draw on the theory of 'practice architectures' [24].

The analysis started with the transcripts being read several times to gain an overall impression of the material and distinguish patterns, variations, and differences in PE teacher's discussions. The intention was to get an initial picture of the visible text through close empirical reading. Second, the selected texts were decontextualized into meaning units that covered the PE teacher's sayings, doings, and relating's that shaped the practice [26]. The meaning units were enabling and constraining aspects that we marked, condensed, and coded. Third, the codes were sorted and compared to identifying and arranged into discourses. Fourth, we identified key concepts in each discourse to highlight the nuance of the discourses (**Table 1**). Quotations from the PE teachers are presented to illustrate the discourses.

Discourse	Key concepts
Technical-rational	An optimistic approach To handle challenges
Participating	Challenges to motivate all pupils Including all pupils
Steering and supporting	Anchoring work Issues with scheduling Principal prioritization Support from principals and colleges

Table 1.
The identified discourses and key concepts in the research circle meetings.

4. Findings

During the analysis, three discourses were identified consisting of key concepts: how the practice architectures enabled and constrained the PE teachers' implementation of PuLH (**Table 1**). The findings are discussed about practice architectures [24] in the following section. In the excerpts, "IP" means interview person and "R" means researcher.

4.1 Discourses visible in research circle meetings

4.1.1 Technical-rational discourse

The *technical-rational discourse* dominated in the first research circle meeting but was also focused at the second meeting. This discourse refers to PE teachers' *optimistic approach* to technical solutions and their *challenges to handle* with them. The technical solutions covered heart rate equipment, maximum heart rate test, and heart rate zone. At the beginning of the research circle meetings, the more experienced PE teachers who had conducted MVPA activities during a more extended time before PuLH started acted as mentors to less experienced ones. Thus, the practice's social-political arrangements [24] enabled the PE teachers to share knowledge as they shared their experiences, received collegial support, and interacted with each other and the researchers. The more experienced PE teacher's optimistic approach to technical solutions influenced the other PE teachers to initially perceive the equipment as indispensable for pupils' MVPA activities. This means that the cultural-discursive arrangements [24] also initially constrained the PE teacher's discussions. Thus, experienced PE teachers' perspectives influence how they talk about PuLH and introduce less experienced PE teachers.

During the discussions in the first research circle meeting, large parts covered the challenges with the technical solutions. The PE teachers discussed the MVPA session's duration and how long the pupils should be in the correct heart rate zone. A joint decision was made in the discussions, i.e., a heart rate zone between 60 and 80%, since the PE teachers saw a risk of not receiving the desired effect if the heart rate was too high or too low. They expressed that it was challenging to get the pupils to be within the correct heart rate zone, i.e., not too high and not too low heart rate, and sometimes pupils' efforts did not seem to match what the heart rate monitor showed. Besides, the PE teachers discussed that some pupils need to get to know their bodies better, and they informed the pupils that it is not dangerous to have a high heart rate. In the first and second research circle meetings, the PE teachers also discussed that they shared experiences regarding difficulties in performing satisfactory maximum heart rate tests among pupils. That was especially difficult among pupils who had poor physical fitness, which can be seen in the following excerpt:

> *IP2: Yes, I agree with the maximum heart rate test, that it is difficult to get the pupils' heart rate up. Many pupils do not have a routine of being out and physically active, and may even feel uncomfortable getting out, as they have not done it before. One thinks they are completely exhausted even though one may not be close to their max... (Research circle meeting 2, afternoon).*

The maximum heart rate test among pupils [38] and the correct heart rate zone were problematized during the meetings due to methodological differences in previous studies (e.g., [39–42]).

At this time in Sweden, there was a societal discussion about MVPA and that these would positively impact pupils' academic performance and grades. The PE teachers' attitude to and discussions about this might have been influenced by cultural-discursive arrangements (cf. [24]), such as this societal discussion and an attentive book [43] within the theme and similar projects at other schools (e.g., [44]). The PE teachers' positive view of MVPA's impact on academic performance and grades might also have been influenced by results from systematic literature reviews, which indicate a relationship between MVPA and increased academic performance [40–42]. This shows that both national and international discourses influence what is possible to say and do in a specific context at a particular time [24]. However, the researchers problematized the evidence of MVPAs impact on academic performance within the research circle meetings since studies show that only one-third of the studies meet the criteria for estimating statical power (e.g., [42]). Likewise, MVPA has a minimal beneficial impact on the pupil's academic performance or even a negative impact [39].

In the PE teachers' discussions in the two first research circle meetings, the PE teachers discussed allowing pupils who have learned to be in the correct heart rate zone to do MVPA without a heart rate monitor.

> *IP4: I think that it is the movement we want, and I notice that they [the pupils] have better movement sometimes; it is ok that not everyone wears a heart rate monitor.*
>
> *IP6: it is also possible to use it in another teaching.*
>
> *IP4: yes exactly, it certainly is not a loss in that way. I think it's a poor argument that it [the heart rate band] should only be for that [MVPA activities].*
>
> *R: it may be good at first, and then later it can be lent out to another school.*
>
> *IP4: yes, exactly. Or some new ones [pupils in grade 7] that are coming.*
>
> *Since perhaps the eighth graders [pupils in grade 8] are already familiar and accustomed to it, it will be a financial saving for them instead of buying new all the time.*
>
> *IP5: they know roughly how they are to be [in the heart rate zone] to...*
>
> *R: they [the pupils] have learned it [the heart rate zone] (Research circle meeting 3 – forenoon).*

In the third research circle meeting, discussions of the importance of technical solutions were no longer dominating. The PE teachers developed knowledge over time in parallel with us presenting and problematizing current research results (e.g., [39–42]) and their experiences of implementing PuLH and the possibility to discuss with each other. The PE teachers discovered that if MVPA can be conducted without a heart rate monitor, it provides an opportunity for them to be outdoor and space for more classes to participate in MVPA. Some schools had a sports hall for MVPA sessions, whereas others were forced to have MVPA sessions in a big lecture hall that was unsuitable for PA. Thus, the material-economic arrangements [24] constrained some of the PE teachers' practices by not having the opportunity to have the PuLH lessons in a sports hall and having a heart rate monitor for all pupils.

4.1.2 Participating discourse

The *participating discourse* occurred within all discussions in the research circle meetings but increased after each meeting and became most dominant in the last meeting. This reflects the content and development of the research circle meetings that included health promotion, a child-centred coaching approach, SDT, and adapted PA.

This discourse covers PE teachers' discussions regarding *challenges to motivate all pupils* and how to handle these by coaching pupils to participate in MVPA. Coaching was something that the PE teachers also applied in the first research circle meeting. Challenges to motivating all pupils were experiences that several PE teachers shared, especially those who seldom participated in ordinary PE.

> *IP5: It is, of course, the pupils who do not go there at all, it is really very difficult. They do not participate in ordinary PE lessons either, etc. //...// We have not really found those pupils that ... we have motivated others, but not them (Research circle meeting 1, forenoon).*

At the first and second research circle meetings, the PE teachers also discussed motivation issues covering some pupils not wanting to participate if they show their bodies in front of peers. They said, for instance, some pupils express discomfort in the locker room when they put on the heart rate monitor since they must expose their bodies in front of peers. This also emerged in the study where we interviewed the pupils in the PuLH intervention [23]. Indeed, some pupils associate PE and MVPA with anxiety and discomfort due to negative self-image and body perception [45]. The social-political arrangements [24] enabled the PE teacher to share the experience of some solutions. For example, some PE teachers expressed that they adapted the locker room situation by motivating the pupils to shower in private such as using shower curtains or having school staff in the locker room. Other PE teachers shared experiences adapting the MVPA activities to include all pupils, such as listening to pupils' voices of their needs so that all could and wanted to participate. The PE teachers also discussed that since the MVPA activities were not graded, it made it easier to *include all pupils* to participate, which also was found in the study with the pupils [23]. In addition, to include all pupils, the PE teachers allowed them to choose activities, which can be seen in the following excerpt:

> *IP1: There is no assessment there at all; there is no one who stands and examines me [the pupils] critically and checks what skills and abilities I have. It's a way of attempting to get them involved. It's just, you should just try to move about more here. And we often have that they get to choose between different activities and that is great because then one chooses something one feels safe and comfortable with (Research circle meeting 1, forenoon).*

To encourage the pupils to participate in the MVPA activities, the PE teachers created individual solutions for pupils with special needs, such as neuropsychiatric disabilities and physical disabilities. For example, they were offering additional MVPA activities each week to make it possible for them to concentrate better in the classroom, which also was found in the study with the pupils [23]. Furthermore, to make it possible for all pupils to want to participate in MVPA activities, they offered some pupils (often girls, pupils with overweight, and immigrants) to enter the locker room earlier to avoid exposing their bodies. The following excerpt illustrates how one PE teacher creates a solution to increase the possibility for pupils with overweight to want to participate:

> *IP2: We have had problems with some finding it uncomfortable to have a heart rate monitor and then having to feel it, having to put on the heart rate monitor in front of others in the locker room if they are perhaps a little overweight, and things like that. So, in such a situation, we have made alternative arrangements available to them; they are not required to wear the heart rate monitors every time; it is better that they still move about ... but they are not connected up [attached] (Research circle meeting 1, forenoon).*

These adjustments align with the content of the research circle meetings in which the PE teachers took part in lectures and workshops on health promotion and health coaching. These activities might explain this adaptation and development of PuLH. The PE teachers received lessons and workshops on adapted PA and health coaching in the research circle meetings to encourage all pupils to participate. In the last research circle meeting, the PE teachers shared the experience that they had adapted the MVPA sessions over time to create opportunities for all pupils to participate. The PE teachers also described that they noticed that the pupils' conflicts had decreased, and cohesion improved. Thus, the cultural-discursive arrangement [24] has enabled the PE teachers to jointly reflect and contribute to shaping the PE teachers' talk about PuLH content and new ways of coaching and knowledge necessary for creating new ways and solutions to develop PuLH activities.

> *R: has your way of working with MVPA changed over time when they have worked with it? //...//.*
>
> *IP1: ... We have put more focus on the fact that they only raise the heart rate. //...// We play more now we did than before. //...//.*
>
> *IP2: Gradually, we have loosened up a bit [the activities] a little more voluntarily. From the beginning, the situation was that everyone does the same things when one stays in the heart rate zone, but then when it gets where one wants it [the pupils feel that they are in the right heart rate zone], they get a little more in terms of alternative options to do something else. I'm going to practice my ballet dance, well then do it. //...// One finds a corner so that they can do it so that they not only stand in front of that board but rather they can ...*
>
> *R: be flexible [?]*
>
> *IP2: yes (research circle meeting 3, afternoon).*

4.1.3 Steering and supporting discourse

The *steering and support discourse* occurred in the discussions in all research circle meetings but dominated, especially in the second meeting. At these meetings, the PE teachers discussed and reflected upon how to progress with the implementation process in their schools. They discussed the importance of conducting school *anchoring work* to involve all school staff. This is a social-political arrangement [24] that enables to carry out the implementation. Another issue within this discourse refers to *issues with scheduling*. PE teachers at some schools discuss that poor scheduling, e.g., short time between MVPA sessions and the following lesson, contributed to a stressful situation for the pupils. Some of the PE teachers in the theoretical subjects were very negative and gave invalid absences to the pupils that arrived a little late.

> *IP3: ...it became very tight in the schedule. The pupils only have ten minutes to change clothes before the MVPA activities //...//. Then after the workout, they have a quarter of an hour to be back in the classroom after showering and changing again...*
>
> *IP4: I can fill in there. We have had the same dilemma with the schedule. The negative impacts are that the colleagues who are connected to the MVPA activities' become very negative and have even started to put invalid absence on the pupils [record], even though they have ten minutes on the schedule to finish and change [clothes] to go to the next lesson (Research circle meeting 2, forenoon).*

The PE teachers in the theoretical subjects have a power position over the pupils, which indicates the importance of clearly anchoring the implementation of PuLH in the schools so that all PE teachers facilitate a good situation for the pupils. The PE teachers discussed the importance of scheduling MVPA carefully to prevent pupils' stress. Some of the pupils in PuLH also expressed that they experienced negative stress due to poor scheduling [23]. The school's decision on how MVPA activities' scheduled is a social-political arrangement [24] that conditions the PE teachers' opportunities to run PuLH. PE teachers at schools who had planned PuLH carefully described that the scheduling between ordinary lessons and PuLH had worked well. The PE teachers also discussed the importance of schedule MVPA before lunch to positively affect the pupils during the whole school day. Similar findings were also found among the pupils in PuLH [23].

The PE teachers discussed the pupils' energy balance, and the need to promote their opportunities to get enough food at school as they became hungry when they were more physically active. Some of the PE teachers describe that the pupils became hungrier after PuLH started; despite this, they were not allowed to eat more lunch because there was no more food available. The limited school lunch constrained the practice and therefore was framed by the material-economic arrangement [24] because the pupils had difficulty coping with the lessons after PuLH if they were hungry. At the same time, this arrangement enables the practice in other schools since the *principals prioritized* and had decided that the pupils were offered refreshments and breakfast to have enough energy to manage the whole school day after introducing PuLH. They have also decided to extend the school week by 90 minutes to reduce stress between lectures. These efforts entail increased costs, and some of the PE teachers described that their school does not have the financial opportunities. In contrast, other PE teachers said that their principal had prioritized it.

> *IP4: it is precisely this comprehensive way of thinking so certain heart rate-boosting activity in all its glory, but then there is a lot of other things in terms of sleep and diet that have an impact and that is how we as a school deal with it? We have extended our school day, unlike some others, because some drive, take a little time from each subject. We have actually extended our school week by 90 minutes, which means that they ended at 10 to 3 at the latest. Now we have those who go to a quarter to four and the days that they go a long time, they also get a snack in the afternoon. So it was also such a thing as after this that we replenish with that energy intake even after lunch.*

> *IP2: it is where we want to be (Research circle meeting 2, forenoon).*

This discourse also involves discussions regarding PE teachers' experience of *support from principals and colleagues* and lack of support. Some PE teachers feel lonely as they do not get enough support and help from other colleagues. In these cases, they would like the principal to mark. Other PE teachers express positive support experiences from their principal, who has communicated that the PuLH-intervention will be conducted. Also, the principal has provided an additional teaching resource. However, some PE teachers described feeling a lack of support from principals due to a lot of responsibility placed on them to do PuLH work. The support is framed by a material-economic arrangement [24] that influences PE teachers' practice opportunities.

Another aspect of this discourse covers that PuLH was arranged so the PE teachers could participate in the research circle meetings and discuss with teachers in the same profession and be free from teaching during the three full-days meetings. This material-economic arrangement [24] of the practice enabled all PE teachers to participate in research circle meetings. In the last research circle meeting, the PE teachers reflected upon the value of taking part in these meetings. The PE teachers discussed that they had learned a lot since they had had the opportunity to discuss with the researchers and support and help each other since they share many similar experiences.

> *IP1: It has been positive, it has been nice to meet others who have also struggled with the same difficulties, or the same issues, and get input on how the leadership stands at different schools. How to solve purely in terms of logistics and scheduling. Getting new thoughts and ideas.*
>
> *IP5: Yes, we have really looked forward to these meetings, to discuss certain things and hear how things should be done and such.*
>
> *IP2: Getting some critical eyes, how can one do that in that way, or what did you think about that there? (Research circle meeting 3, afternoon).*

The social-political arrangements [24] for the meeting practice made it possible for the PE teachers to collaborate and develop the activities. Indeed, a previous study confirms the value of researchers and practitioners working together to develop teachers' actions [18]. Finally, some PE teachers expressed that their school principal had decided that PuLH should become an ordinary part of the school day, which is a material-economic arrangement [24] that enables the PE teachers' implementation of PuLH.

5. Conclusions

When implementing a health-promoting intervention with an influence of a bottom-up approach such as PuLH, the PE teachers' interests, and questions are central, unlike other more traditional top-down programs [46]. However, the implementation of PuLH has been challenging since the implementation is both enabled and constrained by the practice of other PE teachers and principals practices. Challenges often arise when interventions are implemented [2, 3]. The material-economic arrangement [24] shapes the practice visible in the steering and supporting discourse, which meant that all PE teachers were allowed to participate in the research circle meetings and were given enough time aside to implement PuLH. This is essential for PE teachers to be able to run and implement interventions (cf. [3, 15]). In this study, the findings demonstrate that PuLH worked well for the pupils in the schools that provided enough food (refreshments, lunch, and sometimes breakfast) and extended the school day to reduce stress between PuLH and the next lesson. In these cases, PuLH was well-planned and proved to offer equal conditions for all pupils. Indeed, PuLH promoted health and well-being among the pupils [23]. Well-planned health promotion interventions in school should promote pupils' well-being and thus align with the UN Convention on the Rights of the Child (UNCRC) [47]. At the same time, the findings also demonstrate that some PE teachers were given unequal conditions to implement PuLH. For example, a low level of anchoring had been implemented, they had poorer scheduling and received less support from colleagues and principals, which constrained the implementation work. Good conditions in health promotion interventions are essential for teachers to be able to run and implement interventions [2, 3]. However, the discussion in the research circle meetings about contextual factors increased the PE teachers' awareness that structural challenges must reach the principals of schools where this was a problem.

Another conclusion is that the PE teachers' reflections and discussions were shaped by cultural-discursive arrangements (cf. [24]), showing how the PE teachers strengthen each other by willingly sharing experiences and helping each other during the research circle meetings to develop a well-planned PuLH. By sharing experiences, they found out how others dealt with practical issues, and in turn, they could bring new insights to their practice to develop, reflecting the idea within the research circle (i.e., [34, 35]). With PE teachers' interactions and openness in the social intersubjective space [24], the research circle meetings assisted new relationships and collegial support. The PE teachers' professional development might have been influenced by the other teachers' practices and initiatives and their ability to collaborate with the others. In addition, the PE teachers' professional development may have benefited from the collaboration with the researchers when jointly critically reflecting on the implementation of a child-centred perspective on practice. Indeed, researchers can act as catalysts for the discussions within the research circle meetings necessary for teachers' processes and professional development (cf. [15]).

The process of the research circle meetings demonstrated that the PE teachers started to problematize the implementation of PuLH. The PE teachers' new insights and transformed views were shaped by social-political arrangements (cf. [24]). In this arrangement, the technical-rational discourse dominated initially and then decreased during the meetings. The PE teachers took a critical stance, revalued the heart rate equipment, and found new ways of using it by sharing experiences. For instance, the PE teachers became convinced that the heart rate equipment is not needed in the same way and extent. They maintained that it is helpful in the beginning when pupils need to get to know their body and their heart rate. In the participating discourse, it was clear that the PE teachers created solutions to include all pupils in PuLH, for instance, listening to the pupils' voices, adapting the locker-room situations, and tailored solutions for pupils with special needs. The content might explain this solution-oriented approach in the research circle meetings, which focused on a child-centred coaching approach. The participating discourse in this study is also in line with a health promotion practice (cf. [48]).

An action research approach can play an essential role in implementing health-promoting interventions for pupils. In this way, PE teachers are stimulated to participate more actively in the research process than is usual. The researchers helped shape the design of the PuLH, and at the same time, the PE teachers have contributed insights into what works and does not work in practice. Thus, the PE teacher's specific knowledge of their practice is essential since an intervention needs to be implemented within the particular context and their contextual factors [2]. Through this collaboration, theory and practice have intertwined as both parties have contributed with experiences and knowledge that developed PuLH. This has been important to stimulate critically conscious acting and decision-making, which is essential when building coalitions between researchers and practitioners.

Acknowledgements

We are grateful for receiving funding from the Center of research on Welfare, Health and Sport (CVHI), School of Health and Welfare, Halmstad University, and the Department of Research and Development within Education, Region Jönköping County, Sweden, and the participating municipalities in the Region Jönköping.

Conflict of interest

The authors declare no conflict of interest.

Thanks

The authors are grateful to the Directors of Education, the principals, development managers where data collection occurred. We especially thank the PE teachers who participated in the study. We also gratefully acknowledge Yvonne Lindén Andersson, Department of Research and Development within Education, Region Jönköping County, Sweden, for transcribing the recorded discussions during the research circle meetings.

Author details

Linn Håman[1*], Katarina Haraldsson[2,3] and Eva-Carin Lindgren[1]

1 School of Health and Welfare, Halmstad University, Halmstad, Sweden

2 Department of Research and Development Within Education, Halmstad, Sweden

3 School of Public Health and Community Medicine, Institute of Medicine, University of Gothenburg, Gothenburg, Sweden

*Address all correspondence to: linn.haman@hh.se

References

[1] Pearson M, Chilton R, Woods HB, Wyatt K, Ford T, Abraham C, et al. Implementing health promotion in schools: Protocol for a realist systematic review of research and experience in the United Kingdom (UK). Systematic Reviews. 2012;**1**:48. Available from: http://www.systematicreviewsjournal.com/content/1/1/48

[2] Meyers DC, Durlak JA, Wandersman A. The quality implementation framework: A synthesis of critical steps in the implementation process. American Journal of Community Psychology. 2012;**50**:462-480. DOI: 10.1007/s10464-012-9522-x

[3] Darlington EJ, Violon N, Jourdan D. Implementation of health promotion programmes in schools: An approach to understand the influence of contextual factors on the process? BMC Public Health. 2018;**18**:163. DOI: 10.1186/s12889-017-5011-3

[4] Rowling L, Samdal O. Filling the black box of implementation for health-promoting schools. Health Education. 2011;**111**(5):347-366. DOI: 10.1108/09654281111161202

[5] Smith BJ, Tang KC, Nutbeam D. WHO health promotion glossary: New terms. Health Promotion International. 2006;**21**(4):340-345. DOI: 10.1093/heapro/dal033

[6] Swedish Government Official Reports. Forska tillsammans—samverkan för lärande och förbättring. [Research together—collaboration for learning and improvement]. [Internet]. 2018. Available from: https://www.regeringen.se/4933fc/contentassets/1e0e6381c554497ab51eeeb13d36b1ce/sou-2018_19.pdf [Accessed: November 14, 2021]

[7] Elm A, Nordqvist I. The research circle—a tool for preschool teachers' professional learning and preschool development. European Journal of Teacher Education. 2019;**42**(5):621-633. DOI: 10.1080/02619768.2019.1652899

[8] Hilton A, Hilton G, Dole S, Goos M. School leaders as participants in teachers' professional development: The impact on teachers' and school leaders' professional growth. Australian Journal of Teacher Education. 2015;**40**(12):104-125. DOI: 10.14221/ajte.2015v40n12.8

[9] Tam ACF. The role of a professional learning community in teacher change: A perspective from beliefs and practices. Teachers and Teaching: Theory and Practice. 2015;**21**(5):22-43. DOI: 10.1080/13540602.2014.928122

[10] Hargreaves A, Fullan M. Professionellt Kapital - Att Utveckla Undervisning i Alla Skolor [Professional Capital - Transforming Teaching in every School]. Lund: Studentlitteratur; 2016

[11] Sprott RA. Factors that foster and deter advanced teachers' professional development. Teaching and Teacher Education. 2019;**77**:321-331. DOI: 10.1016/j.tate.2018.11.001

[12] Owen KB, Smith J, Lubans DR, Ng JYY, Lonsdale C. Self-determined motivation and physical activity in children and adolescents: A systematic review and meta-analysis. Preventive Medicine. 2014;**67**:270-279. DOI: 10.1016/j.ypmed.2014.07.033

[13] Timperley H. Realizing the Power of Professional Learning. Maidenhead: Open University Press; 2011

[14] Holmstrand L, Härnsten G. Förutsättningar för forskningscirklar i

skolan: en kritisk granskning [Conditions for Research Circles in Schools: A Critical Review]. Stockholm: Authority for School Development; 2003

[15] Fändrik AK, Lundgren M, Nerström N. Kollegial professionsutveckling för skolledare och lärare inom gymnasial yrkesutbildning: En fallstudie av en forskningscirkel [Collegial professional development for school leaders and teachers in upper secondary vocational education: A case study of a research circle]. Nordic Journal of Vocational Education and Training. 2018;**8**(2):1-21. DOI: 10.3384/njvet.2242-458X.18821

[16] Gustafsson P, Jonsson G, Nilsson T. Teknikämnet i svensk grundskolas tidiga skolår sett genom forskningscirkelns lupp [The subject of technology in the early school years of Swedish primary school seen through the loupe of the research circle]. Nordic Studies in Science Education. 2018;**14**(2):113-124

[17] Holmstrand L. Deltagarbaserad aktionsforskning—Ett nytt paradigm? [Participant-based action research—A new paradigm?]. In: Wingård B, editor. Livslång nyfikenhet. En vänbok till Gunilla Härnsten [Lifelong Curiosity. A Friend Book for Gunilla Härnsten]. Stockholm: HSL Publishers; 2006

[18] Wahlgren B, Aarkrog V. Bridging the gap between research and practice: How teachers use research-based knowledge. Educational Action Research. 2021;**29**(1):118-132. DOI: 10.1080/09650792.2020.1724169

[19] The Swedish Ministry for Education. School Act, chapter 1 § 5 [Internet]. 2010, 800. Available from: https://www.riksdagen.se/sv/dokument-lagar/dokument/svensk-forfattningssamling/skollag-2010800_sfs-2010-800 [Accessed: October 10, 2021]

[20] The Swedish Research Council. Forskning och skola i samverkan – Kartläggningar av forskningsresultat med relevans för praktiskt arbete i skolväsendet [Research and school in collaboration—Surveys of research results with relevance for practical work in the school system]. Stockholm; 2015

[21] WHO. Ottawa charter for health promotion. In: First International Conference on Health Promotion. Ottawa: WHO; 1986

[22] Wold B, Mittelmark MB. Health-promotion research over three decades: The social-ecological model and challenges in implementation of interventions. Scandinavian Journal of Public Health. 2018;**46**:20-26. DOI: 10.1177/1403494817743893

[23] Lindgren E-C, Haraldsson K, Håman L. Voices from pupil participation in the health promotion intervention "pulse for learning and health [PuLH]" in primary and middle school. International Journal of Environmental Research and Public Health. 2019;**16**(22):4543. DOI: 10.3390/ijerph16224543

[24] Kemmis S, Grootenboer P. Situating praxis in practice. In: Kemmis S, Smith T, editors. Enabling Praxis: Challenges for Education. Amsterdam: Sense Publishing; 2008. pp. 37-62

[25] Kemmis S. The Action Research Planner Doing Critical Participatory Action Research. Singapore: Springer; 2014

[26] Kemmis S. Action research: A practice-changing practice. Educational Action Research. 2009;**17**(3):313-331. DOI: 10.1080/09650790903093284

[27] Wallace M. A historical review of action research: Some implications

for the education of teachers in their managerial role. Journal of Education for Teaching. 1987;**13**(2):97-115. DOI: 10.1080/0260747870130201

[28] Bergman L. Supporting academic literacies: University teachers in collaboration for change. Teaching in Higher Education. 2016;**21**(5):516-531. DOI: 10.1080/13562517.2 016.1160220

[29] Ardoy DN, Fernández-Rodríguez JM, Jiménez-Pavón D, Castillo R, Ruiz JR, Ortega FB. A physical education trial improves adolescents' cognitive performance and academic achievement: The EDUFIT study. Scandinavian Journal of Medicine and Science in Sports. 2014;**24**:e52-e61. DOI: 10.1111/sms.12093

[30] de Greeff JW, Bosker RJ, Oosterlaan J, Hartman CVE. Effects of physical activity on executive functions, attention and academic performance in preadolescent children: A meta-analysis. Journal of Science and Medicine in Sport. 2018;**21**(5):501-507. DOI: 10.1016/j.jsams.2017.09.595

[31] Rasberry CN, Lee SM, Robin L, Laris BA, Russell LA, Coyle KK, et al. The association between school-based physical activity, including physical education, and academic performance: A systematic review of the literature. Preventive Medicine. 2011;**2**(1):S10-S20. DOI: 10.1016/j.ypmed.2011.01.027

[32] Janssen I, Leblanc AG. Systematic review of the health benefits of physical activity and fitness in school-aged children and youth. International Journal of Behavioral Nutrition and Physical Activity. 2010;**11**(7):40. DOI: 10.1186/1479-5868-7-40

[33] Poitras V, Gray C, Borghese M, Carson V, Chaput J, Janssen I, et al. Systematic review of the relationships between objectively measured physical activity and health indicators in school-aged children and youth. Applied Physiology, Nutrition, and Metabolism. 2016;**41**(6):197-239. DOI: 10.1139/apnm-2015-0663

[34] Härnsten G. Forskningscirkeln – Pedagogiska Perspektiv [The Research Circle—Pedagogical Perspectives]. Stockholm: LO; 1995

[35] Härnsten G. Kunskapsmöten i skolvärlden – Exempel från Tre Forskningscirklar [Knowledge Meetings in the School World – Examples from Three Research Circles]. Stockholm: The Swedish National Agency for Education; 2001

[36] The Swedish Research Council. Good Research Practice [Internet]. 2017. Available from: https://www.vr.se/download/18.5639980c162791bbfe697882/1555334908942/Good-Research-Practice_VR_2017.pdf [Accessed: January 14, 2022]

[37] Graneheim UH, Lindgren BM, Lundman B. Methodological challenges in qualitative content analysis: A discussion paper. Nurse Education Today. 2017;**56**:29-34. DOI: 10.1016/j.nedt.2017.06.002

[38] Gelbart M, Ziv-Baran T, Williams CA, Yarom Y, Dubnov-Raz G. Prediction of maximal heart rate in children and adolescents. Clinical Journal of Sport Medicine. 2017;**27**(2):139-144. DOI: 10.1097/JSM.0000000000000315

[39] Quinto Romani A, Klausen TB. Physical activity and school performance: Evidence from a Danish randomised school-intervention study. Scandinavian Journal of Educational Research. 2017;**61**(4):479-502. DOI: 10.1080/00313831.206.1172498

[40] Bidzan-Bluma I, Lipowska M. Physical activity and cognitive

functioning of children: A systematic review. International Journal of Environmental Research and Public Health. 2018;**15**(4):E800. DOI: 10.3390/ijerph15040800

[41] Donnelly JE, Hillman CH, Castelli D, Etnier JL, Lee S, Tomporowski P, et al. Physical activity, fitness, cognitive function, and academic achievement in children: A systematic review. Medicine and Science in Sports and Exercise. 2016;**48**(6):1197-1222. DOI: 10.1249/MSS.0000000000000901

[42] Santana CCA, Azevedo LB, Cattuzzo MT, Hill JO, Andrade LP, Prado WL. Physical fitness and academic performance in youth: A systematic review. Scandinavian Journal of Medicine and Science in Sports. 2017;**27**(6):579-603. DOI: 10.1111/sms.12773

[43] Hansen A. Hjärnstark: hur motion och träning stärker din hjärna [Brain Strong: How Exercise and Training Strengthen Your Brain]. Stockholm: Fitnessförlaget; 2017

[44] Seger I. Pulshöjande aktiviteter ger bättre betyg visar forskning i Järfälla [Research in Järfälla shows that MVPA Activities Improve Grades] [Internet]. 2018. Available from: https://via.tt.se/pressmeddelande/pulshojande-aktiviteter-ger-battre-betyg-visar-forskning-i-jarfalla?publisherId=1325304&releaseId=3245593 [Accessed: September 12, 2021]

[45] Lunde C. Att känna sig sämst på idrotten [to feel the worst in PE lessons]. In: Dartsch C, Norberg JR, Pihlblad J, editors. De Aktiva Och de Inaktiva - Om Ungas rörelse i Skola Och på Fritid [the Active and the Inactive—About the Movement of Young People in School and in Leisure Time]. Stockholm: The Swedish Research Council for Sport Science; 2017. pp. 123-135

[46] Laverack G. Health Promotion Practice: Power and Empowerment. London: SAGE Publications Ltd; 2004

[47] United Nations. Convention on the Rights of the Child, UN General Assembly Resolution 44/25 on 25 November. New York, NY: United Nations; 1989

[48] Marent B, Forster R, Nowak P. Theorizing participation in health promotion: A literature review. Social Theory and Health. 2012;**10**(2):188-207. DOI: 10.1057/sth.2012.2

Chapter 7

Art Therapy with the Extent of Health Promotion

Songül Mollaoğlu, Mukadder Mollaoğlu and Safiye Yanmiş

Abstract

Health and art disciplines have worked in cooperation for the development of health from past to present. Today's understanding of health requires the integration of concepts, such as creative thinking, intuitive and aesthetic knowledge, spiritual awareness, integration, and maturation, which are extremely important in the development of health. The examination of the process of making and creating art and the development of aesthetic sensations that occur at the end of this process play an important role in both the development of health, the growth and maturation of the individual, and the recovery and repair of illness. Art activities not only support holistic health but also act as a source of motivation for well-being. The inclusion of art in health care services has positive effects on society from the more broad perspective of health professionals, patients, and their families. In this review, the relationship between art and health, which is as old as human history, is discussed in line with the literature review, and the dimension of art in improving health is examined. In addition, in line with the studies carried out, the effects of art therapy on individuals with health problems and art therapy methods are discussed.

Keywords: art therapy, health, health promotion, effects of art therapy, types of art therapy

1. Introduction

While factors such as trade growth, ease of global travel, and technological progress affect health positively, on the other hand, changes in lifestyle, such as especially stress, unhealthy nutrition, and a decrease in physical activity, have caused health to be negatively affected. Besides, factors such as the increase in natural disasters, financial crises, and security threats are other conditions that negatively affect health. Today, the disease burden has increased significantly with the prolongation of a lifetime with the increase of infectious diseases and noncommunicable chronic diseases that have become active again with the effect of mass population movements, such as migration [1, 2].

Parallel to the social developments in this age, the changing necessities of individuals and communities have also changed the perspective on health, so a health-centered care approach that protects, maintains, and improves the health of the individual, family, and society has gained importance today. This understanding is based on enabling the individual to acquire behaviors that will protect and improve their well-being and make the right decisions about their own health [2]. The World Health Organization (WHO) defines health as "not only the absence of disease or disability but also a complete well-being in terms of physical, mental, and social" [3]. Health is a fundamental human right. In the Ottawa Convention, it is emphasized that to be healthy, there must be food, shelter, peace, as well as sufficient economic resources, a coherent ecosystem, and sustainable resources to maintain health. The acceptance of these prerequisites suggests the relationships between factors such as physical environment, economy, lifestyle, and health. These correlates provide a basis for a health holistic approach at the heart of the definition of health promotion [3, 4].

Health promotion is effective in improving the well-being of individuals physically, psychologically, educationally, and professionally, thanks to preventing health problems, encouraging healthy lifestyles, and facilitating access to health services. Besides, health promotion plays an important role in controlling overall health costs and making families, communities, workplaces, and organizations healthier [5]. Today, the health system and all professions serving in this field need to transform their laws and regulations, vocational training, and practices in a way that will help people to reach optimal health, which is defined as complete well-being in terms of physical, mental, social, emotional, and intellectual [6]. This situation maybe mediated through activities, such as lifestyle changes, raising awareness, changing behavior, and creating environments that support healthy behaviors. It is also the process of enabling individuals to increase control over and improve their own health [7]. Many health behaviors and health promotion theories have been adapted from social learning and behavioral theories and applied to epidemiology, biology, and health sciences. Art and creativity were often excluded from them. Nonetheless, today's understanding of health requires the integration of concepts, such as creative thinking, intuitive and aesthetic knowledge, spiritual awareness, integration, and maturation, which are extremely important in the development of health [8]. The examination of the processes of making and creating art and the development of aesthetic sensations that occur at the end of this process play an important role in both the development of health, the growth and maturation of the individual, and the recovery and repair of illness [9, 10]. Art activities not only support holistic health but also act as a source of motivation for well-being. The inclusion of art in health care services has positive effects on society from the more broad perspective of health professionals, patients, and their families [11]. WHO [9] states that art therapy has an important effect on preventing diseases and finding solutions in the management of diseases.

2. The concept of health promotion

The best-known definition of health promotion is the definition in WHO's Ottawa Convention. Health promotion in the Ottawa Convention is stated as "a process that aims to increase people's control on their health and creates opportunities for them to promote their health" [9, 12]. Health promotion is a process that uses biological, environmental, psychological, and physical components to create impacts on health and prevent illness, disability, and premature death through educational-oriented voluntary behavior change activities [12]. The promotion of health occurs by means of being realized comprehensively without considering each other separately of the social, cultural, political, and economic processes in the society. This process aims to change or improve the characteristics, feelings and thoughts, actions of people, as well as to positively change the health behaviors, possessed environmental and economic conditions in the society [1, 6]. Health has entered into the process of radical change and promotion through the awareness-raising of health promotion and the worldwide adoption of the importance of the concept. The common purpose of health policies particular to each country is to increase the number of healthy individuals in society and to promote public health [1, 2]. The main source of promoting health and reaching the targeted community criteria in health is to increase the "protective and preventive" activities, which are qualified as the first step in the health sector [5, 6]. In this context, ways to promote health may be specified as strengthening the health system, empowering the individual, empowering the society, forming healthy society policies and cooperating between sectors in health for implementing, and increasing the capacity to improve health [7]. One of the methods of improving health and empowering the individual can be through art. Art therapy began to be widely used, especially in the rehabilitation works carried out in the second world war. The term "Art Therapy" was first used by Adrian Hill in 1942 when he was teaching painting at the King Edward VII Sanatorium. Expressive art therapy is used for therapy that uses all art disciplines. Therapists practicing the discipline of expressive art therapy mostly determine their own therapy methods by integrating one or more of the limited areas of psychotherapy methods, such as painting therapy, reading therapy, dance therapy, drama therapy, music therapy, poetry therapy, and psychodrama. Since expressionist art therapy is a practice that took shape in the last half of the 20th century, it still continues to develop and continues to expand its scope and definition [8, 13]. People have benefited from art for centuries to eliminate mental and physical ailments and they still continue to use it as a treatment method. Many different cultures have embraced the idea that creative expression can make a powerful contribution to the healing process. Throughout recorded history, painting, stories, dance, and music have been part of people's lives as healing rituals. Considering the physiological and psychological effects of art, many applications have been made as a method specific to the disorder [14]. Art, which is the way people express themselves, is a way of expressing their feelings, thoughts, and ideas with the help of artistic expressions. On this path, there is psychological relaxation, spiritual rest, and emotional calmness. With the materials used while doing this, it enables people to reflect their weakness, stress, and anxiety, in short, their negative feelings or positive feelings in the opposite direction, or what individuals want to tell, with shapes and symbols that they reveal through art [15]. Art therapy is to reveal the creative process by using art materials therapeutically together with an instructor who has received art therapy training to make individuals feel good. With this method, people rediscover their feelings and themselves, express their thoughts, make them question themselves, provide psychological relief, acquire the ability to manage their own behavior, gain skills, develop self-confidence, reduce stress and anxiety levels, and provide satisfaction, relaxation and comfort.

In all known societies in the world since prehistoric and primitive societies, artistic activities, such as temples, houses, painting, sculpture, and weaving, were carried out. Looking at ancient Greece, medicine and art have been accepted as an inseparable whole. It was believed that healing is spiritual as well as physical and this is possible with art. In the kingdom of Apollo, science and art were referred to as an indispensable part of human health as a whole. In other words, art has taken place in social life starting from an early age. Birth, death, marriage, harvest or crop ceremonies, and religious, spiritual and physical healing rituals were intertwined with art. Ancient people made art a part of their lives by singing, dancing, drumming, drawing, or telling stories [13, 15]. In general, art has an important contribution to human health. Since antiquity, music, painting, theater, and similar human creations have had a healing effect not only on sick individuals but also on normal people. Aside from the healing power of art in people with mental disorders, the positive effects it has on the morale of people, in general, have continued throughout human history [8]. Margaret Naumberg made the first definition of art therapy as a profession in America. She defined it in 1915 at the school where she was the principal and started to implement it. The discovery of the therapeutic power of art dates back to the 1940s. Its professional use began in the 1960s. Adrian Hill claimed that the drawings and paintings they made with tuberculosis patients not only allowed them to evaluate time but also allowed people to express their emotions and traumatic experiences. In 1958, the first art therapy course was opened at New York University, which also taught his methods and principles [8, 13, 15].

3. The concept of art therapy

Art has taken place in social life starting from ancient times. Birth, death, marriage, harvest or crop ceremonies and religious, spiritual and physical healing rituals were performed with artistic activities. Ancient people made art a part of their lives by singing, dancing, drumming, drawing, or telling stories [10, 11]. In a general manner, art has an important contribution to human health. Since ancient times, music, drawing, theater, and similar human creations have had a healing effect not only on sick individuals but also on normal people. In other respects, the healing power of art in people with mental disorders, and the positive effects it has on the morale of people, in general, have continued throughout human history [8, 16].

Art therapy has been used as a therapeutic method, which is characterized as a power to increase health and well-being since the beginning of the 21st century [8]. Art therapy, which is defined as the use of art to improve and strengthen the physical, mental, and emotional health of individuals, benefits from the creative, productive, and dynamic effect of art through artistic activities. Accordingly, art therapy is based on the belief that this creative process, which includes artistic self-expression, helps people resolve conflicts and troubles, improve interpersonal skills, reduce stress, manage behavior, increase self-esteem and self-awareness, and gain insight [17]. In other words, it is the use of performing art by professionals, as a developer and therapeutic, for people who experience disease, trauma, or life difficulties, or who only demand personal development. Performing and using art has been validated to overcome art and other traumatic experiences, improve cognitive skills, and increase getting pleasure in life [8, 13, 18].

The American Art Therapy Association defines art therapy as a mental health profession that uses the creative process of making art to heal and enhance the mental, physical, and emotional well-being of individuals of all ages [17]. The American Art Therapy Association considers this process as the process of making art in a professional relationship with individuals who have mental disorders, experience traumatic processes, and are exposed to difficult living conditions. Individuals' awareness can be improved with the process of making art and what is reflected in the art product, and individuals with mental disorders can better cope with the symptoms caused by their illness. The art creation process provides support to clients in terms of increasing cognitive functions and life satisfaction. According to the Canadian Art Therapy Association, art psychotherapy is the use of what the client reflects on the art product to increase mental, physical, and emotional well-being in the creative process.

Art therapy is a means of creating psychological maturation in individuals by benefiting the power of imagination to create insight, integrity, and healing using art materials. Art therapy is a quite successful and effective means of expressing repressed emotions and underlying conflicts through verbal language. Art therapy is a treatment method used in many spiritual, developmental, neurological, mental, and behavioral disorders. Art therapy is a treatment method used in many spiritual, developmental, neurological, mental, and behavioral disorders. Many art therapists agree that the creative process has a healing power itself [8–11]. For example, a Cochrane review looked at the impact of dance/movement therapy on psychological and physical outcomes in people with cancer. It was determined that dance/movement therapy may have beneficial effects on quality of life and somatization [19]. In another study, which included 421 people and examined nine studies, it was determined that music therapy reduced depressive symptoms and anxiety and supported individuals to continue their daily activities [20]. In a study on Alzheimer's disease testing the feasibility and effectiveness of a multidimensional visual arts intervention called Art, Colors, and Emotions therapy (ACE-t), they reported an improvement in the management of behavioral and psychological symptoms in dementia and a significantly higher measured quality of life [21]. In a study conducted on 55 cancer patients, it was found that there was a significant decrease in pain, fatigue, and anxiety levels after art therapy sessions [22]. Ataseven (2018) applied a 10-week art therapy program to schizophrenic patients receiving inpatient treatment, and it was found that it was beneficial in improving symptom profile, subjective well-being, and insight levels in schizophrenic patients who attended the sessions [23]. According to the findings of another study conducted to improve the psycho-emotional and motor skills of the elderly, using dance and theater elements in art therapy is effective in the treatment and rehabilitation of nervous system and musculoskeletal system diseases and injuries of the elderly, getting away from different problems and gaining new skills [24]. Art therapy enables individuals to express themselves creatively using art and to communicate differently with themselves, others, and their reality. The National Institute for Health and Clinical Excellence (NICE) guidelines for psychosis and schizophrenia emphasize that art therapies, including art therapy, improve negative symptoms of psychosis. As a result of the review of 18 articles on the subject, it was determined that art therapy is a useful, meaningful, and acceptable intervention for patients with schizophrenia. For this reason, NICE guidelines recommend art therapy for all patients with schizophrenia, especially for symptom relief [25, 26].

The art therapy process is based on the discovery that our most basic thoughts and emotions are engraved in the subconscious, and that reaching their full expression will be through shapes rather than words. The aim of art therapy is not to eliminate one's fears, anxieties, restlessness, and unhappiness, but to transform these negative emotions into honest expressions using some creative ways and forms [8, 27]. The aims of art therapy are as follows [27]:

1. To resolve after reaching the "I" phenomenon and the trouble by the individual's self-expression, creativity, and ability method, to put the emotions and troubles that are difficult to express verbally on paper through art, and to overcome the

formidable interferences between the specialist and the patient in a safe environment. The patient individual actually draws his troubles.

2. To solve the potential of the individual with natural expressions, the purpose here is to make easy access of the specialist to the troubles and to establish a bridge between the drawn picture, the person who draws, and the specialist. It helps to resolve emotions and thoughts that are formidable to overcome, thanks to therapy.

3. Through this practice, the person has the opportunity to think and compare by experiencing the trouble and emotions the person has experienced over and over again. Thus, a person beholds by relating between the past and the future, and he learns to take the right steps by choosing how he will react in the same situations he will encounter in the future, with the experience he has gotten as a result of his experiences.

4. The most important feature of art therapy is to compare by confronting the emotions and the unconscious subconscious through the active imagination.

The therapeutic functions of art therapy are listed below [8, 23, 28]:

- Art therapy can be used for people with different needs and challenges. By sharing thoughts and feelings through a visual, a person can experience risk-taking in a supportive relationship. Art therapy provides the emotional maturation of the person, increases self-esteem, and provides psychological and social integration.

- Externalizing the experience by creating images and objects makes it possible to talk through the embodied artwork.

- Some clients can control emotions that they cannot cope with through the images and objects they create.

- The symbols created in art therapy and the interpretation of this symbolic content lay the groundwork for self-understanding and emotional development.

- The work of art that emerges in the art therapy process with its color, shape, and stylistic aspects is permanent. The permanence of the artwork – as opposed to the temporary nature of oral expression – enables art therapists and clients, in particular, to follow and reflect on the changes that occur during therapy. It helps build a sense of focus and continuity that can be difficult to maintain in therapy.

4. Health promotion and art therapy

Art therapists offer a creative "helping" environment to their beneficiaries by integrating the types of artistic expression with helping techniques for humans. The inclusion of art therapy in health promotion practices has been known to be beneficial for so long [8, 27, 29]. Findings show that art-based practices are effective in the formation of general well-being and the improvement of mental health [30, 31]. Art practices contribute to the improvement of individuals' health and increase their awareness of themselves and their well-being. According to WHO [9], art contributes significantly to the development of children, the prevention of health-related problems, the provision of quality care, and the formation of health-promoting behaviors. Besides, it may be possible to prevent dementia and aging-specific problems, treat stress, depression, and anxiety, and also prevent situations such as discrimination, social isolation, and loneliness, which are risk factors for mental health with the use of art therapy in health promotion programs. While it is necessary to be at least a literacy level in health education, which is important in the promotion of health, it has contributed to the improvement of individuals' health by overcoming this interference with many practices of art therapy [32].

Art therapy has been used in clinics for more than a century and is professionally maintained. In recent years, the healing effects, benefits, and significant contributions of art to the healing process have been revealed through systematic and controlled studies, and these studies are becoming increasingly common. The art therapy method, which has been proven in Europe and America and later all over the world with scientific studies and data, has been accepted within the framework of Alternative Medicine practices in the CAMBRELLA study carried out within the European Union, in the American National Health Institute and the World Health Organization (WHO) 2014–2023 strategy document [33]. With the development of technology, it is seen that the ways of applying art therapy are diversified today. In recent years, potential possibilities for art therapy have been tried to be developed using digital technology. Interest in digital technology-based studies and applications is increasing day by day. A review was published on this topic, which included 12 studies with more than 400 records scanned. In this review, it was determined that the possibility of sharing images online and applying art therapy digitally increased by art therapists. It also concluded that technology can increase the relevance and reach of art therapy without compromising the core principles of the profession [14]. In another study examining a total of 563 works on art therapy in the visual arts, it was determined that painting, painting, and photography were the most used modalities in the field of visual arts for art therapy purposes. In these studies, it was concluded that art therapy had effects that improve rehabilitation and reduce psychological distress in patients [34]. Different clinical guidelines from the National Institute for Health and Care Excellence (NICE) include art therapy as an indication with recommended evidence. Evidence-based practices related to art therapy are included in different guidelines. The National Institute for Health and Care Excellence (NICE) presents art therapy as an indication with evidence. Nursing Interventions Classification (NIC) has accepted art therapy as a nursing intervention since the beginning of the 21st century [34, 35].

Art therapy can serve as a link through which individuals can explore past and present experiences, review one's life, cope with, adapt to and adapt to age-related changes, and receive support or physical care during an emotional crisis, such as the loss of an organ, memory, or mobility. Art therapy is especially applied in oncology, dementia, and mental care. Oncological patients are one of the patient groups in which art therapies are most frequently used. Kaimal et al. (2019) applied art therapy to cancer patients and their caregivers. In this study, they reported that art therapy demonstrated positive behaviors, such as pleasure, relaxation, and creative problem solving, in cancer patients and caregivers after treatment. Thus, they showed that short-term art interventions can be beneficial for cancer patients and their stressed caregivers [36].

It is stated that symptoms that affect physical integrity, such as pain, are reduced in cancer patients who are treated with art therapy, the psychosocial process is positively affected, and fatigue and anxiety are reduced [36, 37]. Nainis et al. (2016) evaluated the symptoms of patients after art therapy in their study with cancer patients and observed a reduction in eight of the nine symptoms present in the patients [22].

One of the diseases in which art therapy is widely used is dementia. The NICE guideline for dementia (2016) highlights the value of art therapy for different stages and symptoms of dementia, including non-pharmacological treatments. It also discusses the value of interventions that acknowledge the complexity of the situation and address the person as a whole, including their physical, emotional, social, and cognitive processes [37]. Dementia patients often experience neuropsychiatric symptoms that reduce their quality of life. The pharmacological treatment efficacy of these symptoms is limited. People with this diagnosis need treatment that improve neuropsychiatric symptoms and quality of life. Art therapy has been found to be beneficial in dementia as a result of examining the current 45 literature. With the appropriate structure, dementia patients can produce and evaluate visual art. When a few sample art therapy studies were examined, it was observed that patients enjoyed and improved their neuropsychiatric symptoms, social behavior, and self-esteem. The use of art therapy is recommended for Alzheimer's and other dementia disorders. In a study [38], it was found that art therapy had significant effects on improving attention and some other cognitive functions in dementia patients. In addition, it has been revealed that art therapy methods have many benefits, such as reducing behavioral and psychological symptoms in patients with dementia and their caregivers, improving the social skills of patients, and relieving the burden of dementia caregivers. In a study on another neurological problem, it was determined that art therapy improved perceptual symptoms by acting as a restorative behavior training in Parkinson's patients [39].

Art therapy also has different effects on other health problems. For example, it enables people with disabilities to understand and express their emotions through artistic creation and creative thinking, thereby promoting self-awareness, relaxation, confidence, and self-efficacy. Blomdahl et al., (2018) reveal in their study that the patient contributes to more knowledge by deepening the understanding of the importance of talking to himself in an internal dialogue that occurs when the patient participates in the image, art materials, and art-making process [40]. According to Holmqvist et al., (2017), art therapy has proven that there are situations in which an internal change can be observed in patients by affecting consciousness, self-awareness, and ego-strength, which concerns the work in the therapeutic process [41]. On the other hand, Wahlbeck et al., (2018) proved in their study that the therapy acts as a catalyst for the healing process in women using art therapy. Art therapy has been accepted by women, and by creating visible images, they have shared the burdens of fear, gaining hope and self-confidence in the face of their upcoming birth [42].

In a Health Evidence Network synthesis report from the World Health Organization [43], they determined that there is evidence that the arts play an important role in promoting health, preventing a variety of mental and physical health conditions, and treating or managing conditions that occur throughout life.

Different modalities of art therapies, such as visual arts, music therapy, dance therapy, and drama therapy, are also used as complementary treatments for cognitive and psychological disorders of depression, stress, anxiety, or some neurological symptoms that occur with stroke [44]. In addition, art therapy methods are used to reduce the negative effects of chronic diseases, such as diabetes on the individual [45].

Art therapy as a therapeutic process is an interdisciplinary practice that uses art as an expressive process for self-knowledge and expression of conflicts and inner feelings. It is a therapeutic resource that absorbs different knowledge from many disciplines and therefore aims to heal the individual as a whole through processes of self-knowledge and transformation. Studies show that art therapy has significant effects on health promotion. A mixed-method study was conducted to examine the effects of art therapy on smoking cessation in Taiwanese young smokers. The need for smoking, nicotine addiction, self-esteem, self-efficacy, and smoking cessation were examined. Art therapy reduced adolescents' attachment relationships and the need for an ego identity found by smoking together [46]. The intervention also improved participants' self-efficacy, motivated their willingness to draw, and gave them the opportunity to share challenges and befriend others. Art therapy intervention in youth improved self-efficacy and self-esteem [47]. Roy and Manley (2017) conducted a dance and movement session with people in the UK who were recovering from substance abuse. They found that these activities helped establish therapeutic relationships, friendships, and bonds [48]. The value of incorporating arts-based approaches into health promotion programs has long been recognized as beneficial in influencing change. Such approaches have been used in many Australian schools and have been found to improve general well-being and mental health [29]. According to Silva (2019), the cathartic function of painting, the fluidity of the paint, and the energetic movement of the painting liberates and expands consciousness, allowing the elderly to know more about motor coordination, alertness, awakening sensitivity, intuition, creative and creative spirit, themselves and the world, and provides the expansion of perception [49]. In another study, the effect of art therapy on healthy aging was investigated and it was determined that artistic programs increased the quality of life, decreased negative emotions, anxiety, and increased self-esteem [50].

Art and health can meet in effective coping with crisis situations in a region or the world. As a matter of fact, during the COVID-19 pandemic, art therapy methods were used a lot. The World Health Organization and a coalition of cultural partners called for action to mobilize the arts in the fight against isolation, anxiety, and mourning against the mental health crisis caused by the COVID-19 pandemic. Organizations such as University College London, the Tate galleries, Italy's Castello di Rivoli Contemporary Art Museum, England's newly established National Center for Culture and Arts, Hospital Rooms charity and Saudi philanthropic Art Museum have united under the umbrella of the UK's Healing Arts 2021. From 2 to 26 March, these organizations and the UK's National Center for Culture and Arts arranged weekly virtual meetings and events [51]. In addition, the event "Visions And Voices Of A Healthy Planet: The Healing Arts for World Health Day 2022" drew attention to human-induced climate change. It was emphasized that this climate change poses a threat to the survival of people. It was also stated that climate change significantly changed people's understanding of their own health, well-being, and place in the world. For this purpose, events, where health professionals and artists came together in times of crisis, were organized. To this end, Christopher Bailey, the Art and Health leader of the World Health Organization, headquartered in Geneva, Switzerland, focuses on mobilizing the global media to support the health benefits of art in everyday life. On the other hand, they are mapping the evidence for the physical, mental, and social health benefits of arts and art therapies for the World Health Organization, with a commission from the New York University (NYU) Creative Arts Therapies Consortium and the International Research Alliance [52].

5. Art therapy techniques

People have benefited from art for centuries to eliminate mental and physical ailments and they still continue to use it as a treatment method. Many different cultures have embraced the idea that creative expression can make a powerful contribution to the healing process. Throughout recorded history, painting, stories, dance, and music have been part of people's lives as healing rituals. Considering the physiological and psychological effects of art, many applications have been made as a method specific to the disorder. As explained below, many ideas have been put forward and studies have been made about the contribution of art to the healing process [53]. In the art therapy process, in addition to applying the expression of only one of the different art branches, it is possible to switch from one art branch to another with an intermodel expressive approach. Major art therapy techniques are music therapy, dance therapy, poetry therapy, visual arts therapy, and drama therapy.

5.1 Music therapy

This method is also a method that has been used since ancient times, shamanism. It is a widely used therapy method in the world and especially in our country. "Music has influenced people by creating a trance and time has directed the masses. Because especially music has a feature that intensifies emotions, it has been used as a quite common method in many civilizations to strengthen religious feelings and to treat diseases [8, 54]. The music therapist helps basically treat the patient's health by reaching the treatment methods and goals through using their musical experiences (improvisation, singing, lyricising, listening and discussing music, and moving with music) in various fields, such as cognitive functions, motor skills, emotional and effective development, behavior and social abilities, and quality of life [55]. Music therapy involves using music in a therapeutic relationship to address clients' physical, emotional, cognitive, and social needs. Music therapy, according to the World Federation of Music Therapy [54], is defined as "the use of music and/or musical elements (sound, rhythm, melody, and harmony) to develop and increase the communication, relationship, learning, expression, mobilization, organization, and the other related therapeutic effectiveness, which they need, after designed by a trained music therapist for the purpose of physical, emotional, social, and cognitive requirements of one person or a group." Music therapy provides different ways of communication for people who have difficulty expressing themselves with words. Research on music therapy has demonstrated the effectiveness of treatment by focusing on many areas,s such as general physical rehabilitation, increasing motivation for treatment compliance, providing emotional support to clients and their families, and providing an outlet for the expression of emotions [15, 27, 53].

In the early 1800s, music was used as a therapeutic practice to maintain and improve comfort, and music therapy was defined as a part of the healing process. In the literature, it has been emphasized that music therapy affects individuals positively by establishing a connection between their physical and cognitive characteristics. In many studies, it was found that music therapy has positive effects on health. In the meta-analysis study of Amaral et al. [55], it was found that music lowers blood pressure. In the study by Ekinci and Gökalp [56], it has been found that music therapy reduces the effect of the neuroendocrine response to stress. In the study of Zander et al. [57], it was found that the psychological and physiological health of university students who took music education for 2 years improved and the students showed healthy behaviors. In another study, it was concluded that music strengthens the body's immune system and reduces stress level [58]. In addition, it has been reported in the literature that music therapy supports neuroplasticity in functional brain network organization [59].

Bradt et al (2021) published the results of a review called music interventions for improving psychological and physical outcomes in people with cancer. This study included 81 studies with 5576 participants. Of the 81 studies, 74 included adults and seven included children. This systematic review showed that, compared to standard care, music interventions can have beneficial effects on anxiety, depression, hope, pain, and fatigue in adults with cancer. It was concluded that music therapy, but not music medicine interventions, can improve adult patients' quality of life and fatigue levels [60]. A meta-analysis of nine studies with a total of 421 people from any age group (adolescents to the elderly) found that music therapy was more effective than standard therapy alone. In this study, it was determined that music therapy reduced depressive symptoms and anxiety and helped to improve functioning as well as maintaining participation in work, activities, and relationships [61].

5.2 Film therapy

In movie group therapy, the film or documentary selected by the specialist is watched and discussed and commented on it with the specialist. The people who watch the movie talk about the characters of the movie among themselves, identify with them, and reveal their similar emotions. Thus, individuals experience a non-verbal relief, seriously dwell on the troubles and the causes they watch and think about the measures they can take to solve their troubles by establishing a connection between these and their own troubles, starting from the solutions in the movie. While the synthesis and the discussion of the movie are made, the troubles that are engraved in the subconscious of the individual unwittingly arise [31, 62].

It has been reported in the literature that important learning environments for health promotion can be created by using film therapy [63]. In a study conducted with 24 elderly people, it was found that film therapy had positive effects on happiness and quality of life in elderly individuals. Similarly, another study states that film therapy is an important approach to improve the health of the elderly [36]. It was contributed significantly to the promote the health of individuals with a movie therapy practice organized with 15 young women doing the sex trade. Together with this practice, it was observed that women's sense of branding decreased and there were positive changes in the personal and professional lives of individuals [62]. In a study conducted in the United States, movie therapy was applied to enable schooled youth to have healthy sexual intercourse and to promote health in this direction. As a result of the study, it was reported that young people developed positive knowledge, attitude, and behavior toward sexuality [64].

5.3 Visual art therapy

Visual art is a field that allows people to reveal their journeys to their inner worlds with lines and colors. This expressive feature of visual arts helps individuals to discover themselves and develop their inner perceptions. These non-verbal and expressive supports enable people to be treated psychologically. This functional dimension of visual arts serves as a bridge established in the field of health [8, 17]. The American

Art Therapy Association, which carries out studies on art therapy and health, has defined visual art therapy as helping individuals develop interpersonal skills in solving conflicts or individual troubles, directing behavior, reducing stress, increasing self-worth and individual awareness, and self-realization of the individual [17]. Visual art therapy is performed with dry paint, such as pastel and colored pencils; wet paint, such as gouache, marbling, oil paint, and acrylic; sculpture materials, such as play dough, clay, wire, and colored papers, that can be used for assemblage and collage; and art materials that can be prepared with recyclable wastes collected from the environment [65, 66].

Visual art therapy works with a therapist to gain awareness with the expressions that the individual creates, to cope with anxiety, depression, trauma or chronic diseases, and build self-confidence. With the use of lines and colors in visual art therapy, the person transfers his inner world to paper and works with the emotions conveyed by the therapist. The product embodied gains meaning in the therapeutic intermediate area, accompanied by the therapist. The supportive relationship of the therapist plays an important role in the meaning-making process. The unconscious material symbolized by the picture strengthens the ego [66]. In the literature, a study was conducted on women to improve breast health by using the visual art therapy method. As a result of the study, it was found that visual art is an innovative and quite suitable approach to improving breast health [65]. It was found that the stress and anxiety levels of the caregivers decreased, their positive emotions increased, and their satisfaction with handmade arts improved during the 6-month visual art therapy intervention, which was conducted with the caregivers of cancer patients. Besides, it has been reported that positive communication between caregivers, individuals with cancer, and health professionals has increased by means of visual art therapy [67]. The visual art therapy method was used in the prevention of sexually transmitted diseases through health education among high school youth. At the end of the study, it was concluded that visual art therapy is an innovative method to engage young people and that individuals' knowledge and attitudes toward preventing hepatitis and HIV have increased [68]. In another study, it was reported that visual art therapy practiced with old persons helps individuals to age healthy and increases their well-being and quality of life [69]. Visual art therapy was included in health promotion practices, and as a result, it was observed that students' awareness of health behaviors and their level of well-being increased in his study that Mckay and McKenzie conducted for school-age students [29].

5.4 Dance therapy

The feature of dance as an integrative and healing art dates back to ancient cultures. Dance therapy is a psychotherapy method that helps the individual's social life and physical and emotional development [70]. Dance therapy, according to the definition of Dance and Movement Psychotherapy Institution [71], is the experience of the individual's personal, emotional, physical, and social development and awareness of art within the framework of a creative process with the psychotherapeutic practice of movements and dance. The basis of dance therapy is based on the principle that a person's movements reflect his thought system and emotions. As a result of perceiving and recognizing the movements of the person and expanding the movement repertoire, the dance therapist who witnesses this process helps to increase the awareness of the person, create new movement perceptions, and thus develop new communication mechanisms in their emotions and verbal communication [70].

In one study, healthy women aged 50 years and older were given a 15-week jazz dance program once a week, and significant improvements were observed in the static balance of women as a result of the study [72]. In another study using the Profile of Mood States (POMS) in people with dementia, POMS was administered to 36 people with dementia. POMS was applied to individuals with dementia before and after four therapeutic creative dance sessions, and the scores were analyzed. After the therapeutic creative dance sessions, the patients' stress, depression and confusion decreased, the vitality factor increased significantly. Thus, it was concluded that therapeutic creative dance can provide emotional benefits to dementia patients [73]. In another study, it was found that individuals reached a higher range of motion and knee torque values, and therefore, the risk of falling of individuals decreased with the low-impact dance program performed with 26 middle-aged and old individuals [74]. In the study of Kim et al. [75], a 3-month health promotion program was conducted with old individuals to examine changes in health behaviors, cardiovascular risk factors, and life satisfaction. It has been reported that Korean traditional dance figures practiced by elderly individuals for 3 months are effective in improving health behaviors, increasing life satisfaction, and reducing cardiovascular risk factors in the study. A Greek traditional dance program was practiced for 24 weeks in the study conducted with women with 27 breast cancer survivors. In the study, it was found that dance could be an alternative physical activity option for breast cancer survivors and could provide significant improvements in strength, physical function, and mood [76]. In the study of Argiriadou et al. [77], a Greek traditional dance program was practiced by middle-aged women. It has been concluded that dance significantly improved the subjective health of middle-aged women in the study.

Combining science and art, psychoballet makes use of artistic activities, such as dance, ballet, and theatre. It is aimed to improve the quality of life of people with psychiatric problems or people with disabilities, through artistic activities, such as dance and ballet, and they are rehabilitated, thus helping them to integrate with society and not be socially disconnected. With psychoballet, its effectiveness has been confirmed in people with body image and eating disorders, chronic diseases (human immunodeficiency virus (HIV)/acquired immunodeficiency syndrome (AIDS) and breast cancer), fibromyalgia, and people with disabilities [78].

In another study, Cernuda and Andrés (2019) studied the benefits of Cuban psychoballet in Alzheimer's patients. In this study, psychobalding by Alzheimer's patients had effects such as delaying neurodegeneration and recovering cognitive memories in them [79]. The results of this study revealed that psychobalene is an important and useful non-pharmacological method in patients with Alzheimer's and other dementias.

5.5 Drama therapy

The aim of drama therapy is to show the emotions, thoughts, and characters undertaken in the closest possible way to reality. Individuals are offered the opportunity to judge their own emotions and thoughts and the events they experience from a different perspective [8, 80]. It has been proven that theater is a quite effective and enjoyable practice in promoting health, developing healthy lifestyle behaviors, and strengthening positive health perceptions in the literature [18, 80]. The content of theatrical production in any drama therapy aimed at improving health should be prepared by taking into account the knowledge, attitudes, and behaviors of individuals. In the content, the situations that prevent individuals from changing their behavior should be analyzed and this area should be especially focused on. Individuals to ask questions, discuss, and being allowed for role play about the current trouble enables them to experience behavioral change toward these troubles with this therapy method [32]. In drama therapy, especially socially isolated and shy individuals open up, and the importance they attach to group values and interpersonal relationships begins to increase. Since the client knows that he is pretending, he gets rid of the anxiety caused by revealing himself. Even if individuals pretend, they will start to be themselves after a while, so the problems and conflicts they experience outside begin to be seen during the game. Drama therapy is a very useful method in both diagnosis and treatment. It also has significant effects on older individuals.

In one study, an intergenerational theater group was formed of older adults and university students. As a result of the study, it was reported that the theater improved intergenerational relations and age discrimination decreased. Besides, it has been reported that this practice contributes to the development of health by helping to build self-esteem and confidence, and the development of empathy, social justice, and support feeling between university students and older adults [81]. In Wimpenney's study [82], a theater group was formed from individuals over 50 years of age. It has been stated that this practice provides healing to the health and well-being of individuals. Drama therapy was performed with individuals 6 and 7-year-old in the literature. As a result of the therapy, it was observed that the children began to speak fluently, their mental lexicon improved, and their creativity and concentration increased. Moreover, children's self-confidence and motivation have increased and their communication skills have improved, thanks to this practice [80].

5.6 Poetry therapy

Poetry therapy, based on the healing power of words, offers unique opportunities for individuals to improvise and exhibit creative behaviors. Poetry has a healing power in itself; therefore, it is used efficiently and effectively for the purpose of establishing therapeutic relationships with individuals. Reading and writing poetry positively affect both the personal and interpersonal aspects of the individual. Poetry therapy contributes to becoming clear in the individual's perception of himself and others; increased creativity, self-confidence, and self-expression skills; relieving stress by putting intense emotions on paper; creating new meanings by synthesizing new ideas, insights, and information; to the development of mature coping skills that will enable change in behavior and attitudes [8, 11, 83]. Poetry is used as a tool for the expression of emotions that are difficult to express. This method allows individuals to express themselves, increase self-awareness, help individuals understand their own world, redefine their situations by opening new ways of perceiving reality, and enable therapists to gain deeper knowledge about their clients.

It has been proven that poetry therapy is important for end-stage individuals receiving palliative care treatment, their caregivers, and health professionals in a study in the literature. In this study, it was determined that the feeling of loneliness was reduced and the quality of personal care increased with poetry treatment [11]. It is stated the importance of using poetry therapy by health professionals in a health promotion program for health education in another study [83]. In another study, it was reported that poetry therapy is an effective method to eliminate the loneliness in society and to establish social interaction between individuals during pandemic periods [84].

5.7 Mandala

Mandala is a circle consisting of geometric or organic forms, starting with a point and continuing indefinitely. In nature, sunflowers, tree trunks, and animal patterns, many examples can be seen. Man-made mandalas reflect symbols of eastern and western cultures that have different meanings together. In art therapy, the mandala has a different place because it helps to heal and develops consciousness. Starting with a point in the center and continuing, this technique grows as you draw, creating a meditative effect on individuals. It relaxes them, relaxes them, increases creativity and individual awareness. Mandala is a method of concentration. While drawing, all attention should be given to the drawn lines. Thus, it is ensured that the person stays in the moment. This helps the person to keep himself away from stress, worry, and anxiety [53]. Mandala making in art therapy is used to help patients feel at the center of their lives, to express themselves, and to help people discover who they are in the group [85].

6. Conclusion

As a result, the increase in communicable diseases and noncommunicable chronic diseases has provided preventive and preventive studies gain importance. This situation reveals the necessity of integrating art therapy into health promotion practices. By means of integrated art-based approaches, individuals gain and maintain health-promoting knowledge, attitudes, and behaviors. In this study, it has been proven that healthy life and well-being for individuals of all ages, which is the main purpose of health promotion programs, is possible with art therapy practices. Despite the critical importance of art therapy in the health promotion program, studies on this field in the literature are insufficient. Therefore, health professionals and disciplines in the field of art should direct their work together, and increase the health and well-being of society by increasing the evidence on this subject.

Acknowledgements

This research received no specific grant from any funding agency in the public, commercial, or not-for-profit sectors.

Conflict of interest

The authors declare no conflict of interest.

Author details

Songül Mollaoğlu[1], Mukadder Mollaoğlu[2] and Safiye Yanmış[3*]

1 Painting Business Education, Faculty of Education, Department of Fine Arts Education, Sivas Cumhuriyet University, Sivas, Turkey

2 Faculty of Health Science, Sivas Cumhuriyet University, Sivas, Turkey

3 Faculty of Health Science, Erzincan Binali Yıldırım University, Erzincan, Turkey

*Address all correspondence to: safiyeyanmis61@gmail.com

References

[1] Aydın N. Health promotion. Black Sea Journal of Health Science. 2019;**2**:21-29

[2] Kumar S, Preetha G. Health promotion: An effective tool for global health. Indian Journal of Community Medicine. 2012;**37**(1):5-12

[3] Larson JS. The World Health Organization's definition of health: Social versus spiritual health. Social Indicators Research. 1996;**38**(2):181-192

[4] Sartorius N. The meanings of health and its promotion. Croatian Medical Journal. 2006;**47**(4):662-664

[5] Değerli H, Yiğit A. Determination of the healthy lifestyle behavior level of individuals in health protection and health promotion. Süleyman Demirel University Visionary Journal. 2020;**11**(27):573-586

[6] Şimşek Z. The history and strategies based on the samples of health promotion. TAF Preventive Medicine Bulletin. 2013;**12**(3):343-358

[7] Özvarış ŞB. Health promotion and health education. In: Güler Ç, Akın L, editors. Public Health Basic Knowledges. Ankara: Hacettepe University Publications; 2012. pp. 1676-1753

[8] Kahraman ME, Bostancıoğlu B. Art therapy method and techniques health – Effects on improvement power. Journal of Beykoz Academy. 2017;**5**(2):150-162

[9] World Health Organization. Arts and Health [Internet]. 2021. Available from: https://www.who.int/initiatives/arts-and-health [Accessed: October 20, 2021]

[10] Hemingway A, Crossen-White H, Norton E. Using the arts: Learning from a community consultation on health and wellbeing. British Journal of Healthcare Management. 2018;**24**(8):395-403

[11] Gilmour F, Riccobono R, Haraldsdottir E. The value of poetry therapy for people in palliative and end of life care. Progress in Palliative Care. 2020;**28**(1):6-13

[12] World Health Organization. Health Education: Theoretical Concepts, Effective Strategies and Core Competencies. Washington: NLM Classification; 2012

[13] Dalley T, Case C. The Handbook of Art Therapy. London: Routledge; 2014

[14] Zubala A, Kennell N, Hackett S. Art therapy in the digital world: An integrative review of current practice and future directions. Frontiers in Psychology. 2021. DOI: 10.3389/fpsyg.2021.600070

[15] Demir V. Group Psychotherapy in Schizophrenia: Comparison of the Effectiveness of Art Therapy and Mindfulness-Based Cognitive Therapy Programs. Institute of Social Sciences: Üsküdar University; 2021

[16] Aydin B. Medical art therapy. Urrent Approaches in Psychiatry. 2012;**4**(1):69

[17] American Art Therapy Association. About Art Therapy 2009. 2009. Available from: https://arttherapy.org/about-art-therapy/ [Accessed: March 5, 2022]

[18] Chang W-L, Liu Y-S, Yang C-F. Drama therapy counseling as mental health care of college students. International Journal of Environmental Research and Public Health. 2019;**16**(19):3560

[19] Bradt J, Shim M, Goodill SW. Dance/movement therapy for improving psychological and physical outcomes in cancer patients. Cochrane Database of Systematic Reviews. 2015;**1**:CD007103

[20] Aalbers S, Fusar-Poli L, Freeman RE, Spreen M, Ket JCF, Vink AC, et al. Music therapy for depression. Cochrane Database of Systematic Reviews. 2017;**11**:CD004517

[21] Savazzi F. Art, colors, and emotions treatment (ACE-t): A pilot study on the efficacy of an art-based ıntervention for people with Alzheimer's Disease. Frontier in Psychology. 2020;**11**:1467

[22] Nainis N, Paice L, Ratner J, et al. Relieving Symptoms in cancer: Innovaite use of art therapy. Jpain Symptom Management. 2016;**31**:162-169

[23] Ataseven E. The Effects of Art Therapy and Mindfulness-Based Cognitive Behavioral Therapy Applications on Symptom Profile, Insight and Social Functioning in Chronic Schizophrenia Patients Inpatients in Chronic Services. İstanbul: TC Sağlık Bakanlığı Bakırköy Dr. Sadi Konuk Eğitim ve Araştırma Hastanesi; 2018

[24] Paskaleva R, Uzunova A. Role of art therapy for psycho-emotıonal and physical stimulation of the elderly. Research in Kinesiology. 2015;**43**(2):239-241

[25] NICE. Psychosis and schizophrenia in adults: The NICE guideline on treatment and management. NICE Clinical Guideline 178. 2014. https://www.nice.org.uk/guidance/cg178/evidence/full-guideline-490503565 [Accessed March 12, 2022]

[26] Attard A, Larkin M. Art therapy for people with psychosis: A narrative review of the literature. The Lancet Psychiatry. 2016;**3**(11):1067-1078

[27] Işık S. Usage of Pictorial Language in Art Therapy Method and Interpretation of Explanation Forms. Antalya: Akdeniz University; 2013

[28] Edwards D. Art Therapy. Chicago: Sage. Publications; 2014

[29] McKay FH, McKenzie H. Using art for health promotion: Evaluating an in-school program through student perspectives. Health Promotion Practice. 2018;**19**(4):522-530

[30] Oepen R, Gruber H. An art therapy project day to promote health for clients from burnout self-help groups - an exploratory study. PPmP - Psychotherapie Psychosomatik Medizinische Psychologie. 2013;**64**(07):268-274

[31] Hosseini FS, Khodabakhshi-koolaee AT, D. Effectiveness of group film therapy on happiness and quality of life among elderly adults of Kahrizak nursing home. Journal of Health Literacy. 2016;**1**(2):109-117

[32] Mbizvo E. Essay: Theatre—A force for health promotion. Lancet. 2006;**368**:30-31

[33] WHO Traditional Medicine Strategy: 2014-2023. https://www.who.int/publications/i/item/9789241506096 [Accessed April 12, 2022]

[34] Rodriguez Novo N, Novo Muñoz MM, Cuellar-Pompa L, Rodriguez Gomez JA. Trends in research on art therapy indexed in the web of science: A bibliometric analysis. Frontiers in Psychology. 2021;**10**:1-10. DOI: 10.3389/fpsyg.2021.752026

[35] Vaartio-Rajalin H, Santamäki-Fischer R, Jokisalo P, Fagerström L. Art making and expressive art therapy in adult health and nursing care: A scoping

review. International Journal of Nursing Sciences. 2021;**8**(1):102-119

[36] Kaimal G, Councill T, Ramsey K, Cottone C& Snyder K. A conceptual framework for approaches to art therapy research in paediatric hematology/ oncology settings. Canadıan Art Therapy Assocıatıon Journal. 2019;**32**(2):1-9

[37] NICE. Dementia: Supporting people with dementia and their carers in health and social care. 2006. www.nice.org.uk/ guidance/cg42 2006. Last updated 2016; Vol. 42

[38] Wang QY, Li DM. Advances in art therapy for patients with dementia. Chinese Nursing Research. 2016;**3**(3):105-108

[39] Cucca A, Acosta I, Berberian M, Lemen AC, Rizzo JR, Ghilardi MF, et al. Visuospatial exploration and art therapy intervention in patients with Parkinson's disease: An exploratory therapeutic protocol. Complementary Therapies in Medicine. 2018;**40**:70-76

[40] Blomdahl C, Wijk H, Guregård S, ve Rusner, M. Meeting oneself in inner dialogue: A manual-based Phenomenological Art Therapy as experienced by patients diagnosed with moderate to severe depression. The Arts in Psychotherapy. 2018;**59**:17-24

[41] Holmqvist G, Roxberg Å, Larsson I, Ve Lundqvist-Persson C. What art therapists consider to be patient's inner change and how it may appear during art therapy. The Arts in Psychotherapy. 2017;**56**:45-52

[42] Wahlbeck H, Kvist LJ, Landgren K. Gaining hope and self-confidence—An interview study of women's experience of treatment by art therapy for severe fear of childbirth. Women and Birth. 2018;**31**(4):299-306

[43] WHO Regional Office for Europe. Fact sheet - what is the evidence on the role of the arts in improving health and well-being in the WHO European Region? http://www.euro.who.int/__data/assets/pdf_file/0020/412535/WHO_2pp_Arts_Factsheet_v6a.pdf?ua=1 (2019), [Accessed April 11, 2022]

[44] Jang SH, Lee JH, Lee HJ, Lee SY. Effects of mindfulness-based art therapy on psychological symptoms in patients with coronary artery disease. Journal of Korean Medical Science. 2018;**33**:e88. DOI: 10.3346/jkms.2018.33.e88

[45] Tang Y, Li L, Yang Q, Shao Q, Xu Q, Shi H. Art therapy alleviates the levels of depression and blood glucose in diabetic patients: A systematic review and meta-analysis. Frontier in Psychology. 2021;**12**:639626. DOI: 10.3389/fpsyg.2021.639626

[46] Hong R, Guo S, Huang C, Yin C. Examining the effects of art therapy on reoccurring tobacco use in a Taiwanese youth population: A mixed-method study. Substance Use & Misuse. 2017;*53*(4):548-558

[47] Adams C. Group art activities and arts therapies for people using substances: A rapid review of the literatüre. Nordic Journal of Arts, Culture and Health. 2019;**1**(1):47-59

[48] Roy A, Manley J. Recovery and movement: Allegory and 'Journey' as a means of exploring recovery from substance misuse. Journal of Social Work Practice. 2017;**31**(2):191-204

[49] Silva CAM. Contribuição da Arteterapia para a deficiência física. Revista Gestão Educacional. 2019;**12**(12):29-35

[50] Kim SK. A randomized, controlled study of the effects of art therapy on

older Korean-Americans healthy aging. Arts Psychother. 2013;**40**(1):158-164

[51] McGivern H. World to launch global campaign confronting mental health toll of pandemic. The Art Newspaper (ePaper). 2021. https://www.theartnewspaper.com/2021/03/17/world-health-organization-joins-art-world-to-launch-global-campaign-confronting-mental-health-toll-of-pandemic

[52] Visions and voices of a healthy planet: A Healing Arts event for World Health Day 2022. https://www.who.int/news-room/events/detail/2022/04/05/default- calendar/visions-and-voices-of-a-healthy-planet-a-healing-arts-event-for-world-health-day-2022 (Erişim Tarihi:09.04.2022)

[53] Bilgin E. In the process of art therapy treatment of cancer qualıty of lıfe of patıents takıng chemotherapy effect. Isparta: Süleyman Demirel University; 2019

[54] The World Federation of Music Therapy. What is music therapy? [Internet]. 2011. Available from: https://wfmt.info/wfmt-new-home/about-wfmt/ [Accessed: October 12, 2021]

[55] Amaral MAS, Neto MG, de Queiroz JG, Martins-Filho PRS, Saquetto MB, Carvalho VO. Effect of music therapy on blood pressure of individuals with hypertension: A systematic review and Meta-analysis. International Journal of Cardiology. 2016;**214**:461-464

[56] Ekinci M, Gökalp K. Effect of music therapy on anxiety and sleep quality of geriatric haematological oncology patients. The Turkish Journal of Geriatrics. 2020;**23**(4):546-554

[57] Zander MF, Voltmer E, Spahn C. Health promotion and prevention in higher music education: Results of a longitudinal study. Medical Problems of Performing Artists. 2010;**25**(2):54-65

[58] Le Roux FH, Bouic PJD, Bester R. The Effect of choral music on emotions, ımmune parameters and lung function during physiotherapy treatment of pneumonia and bronchitis. South African Journal of Physiotherap. 2007;**63**(2):20-26

[59] Torun Ş. Music based ınterventions in health care: Music therapy, music medicine and others. In: Torun Ş, editor. Music Therapy, Music Medicine and Other Music-Based Practice. 1nd ed. Ankara: Turkish Clinics; 2020. pp. 9-19

[60] Bradt J, Dileo C, Myers-Coffman K, Biondo J. Music interventions for improving psychological and physical outcomes in people with cancer. Cochrane Database of Systematic Reviews. 2021;**10**(10):CD006911

[61] Aalbers S, Fusar-Poli L, Freeman RE, Spreen M, Ket JCF, Vink AC, et al. Music therapy for depression. Cochrane Database of Systematic Reviews. 2017;**11**:CD004517. DOI: 10.1002/14651858.CD004517.pub3

[62] Kendrick C, MacEntee K, Flicker S. Exploring audience engagement and critical narrative ıntervention with the celling sex film. Health Promotion Practice. 2021;**22**(Suppl.2):33-43

[63] Strong P, Lotter G. Reel help for real life: Film therapy and beyond. HTS Teologiese Studies/Theological Studies. 2015;**71**(3):1-8

[64] Brooks-Gunn J, Paikoff RL. Sex is a gamble, kissing is a game: Adolescent sexuality and health promotion. In: Millstein SG, Petersen AC, Nightingale EO, editors. Promoting the Health of Adolescents: New Directions

for the Twenty-first Century. Great Britain: Oxford University Press; 1993. pp. 180-208

[65] Thomas B, Marshall RS, Gold Smith SB, Forrest A. Visual art and breast health promotion: Artists' perspectives. Canadian Oncology Nursing Journal. 2004;**14**(4):233-237

[66] Malchiodi CA. The Art Therapy Sourcebook. New York: McGraw-Hill Companies; 2007

[67] Walsh SM, Martin SC, Schmidt LA. Testing the efficacy of a creative-arts intervention with family caregivers of patients with cancer. Journal of Nursing Scholarship : An Official Publication of Sigma Theta Tau International Honor Society of Nursing. 2004;**36**(3):214-219

[68] Edmondson BJ. Tell me what you see: An arts-based health education program for youth. Health Promotion Practice. 2021;**22**(1):27S-30S

[69] Kim SK. A randomized, controlled study of the effects of art therapy on older Korean-Americans' healthy aging. The Arts in Psychotherapy. 2013;**40**(1):158-164

[70] Sivvas G, Batsiou S, Vasoglou Z, Filippou DA. Dance contribution in health promotion. Journal of Physical Education and Sport. 2015;**15**(3):484-489

[71] Association for Dance Movement Psychotherapy UK. What is Dance Movement Psychotherapy? [Internet]. 2021. Available from: https://admp.org.uk/what-is-dance-movement-psychotherapy/ [Accessed: October 15, 2021]

[72] Wallmann HW, Gillis CB, Alpert PT, Miller SK. The effect of a senior jazz dance class on static balance in healthy women over 50 years of age: A Pilot Study. Biological Research for Nursing. 2009;**10**(3):257-266

[73] De Andrés AL, Pérez E, Cernuda A, Sánchez R. Psychometric properties of Profile of Mood States (POMS) in people with dementia and its application in the evaluation of the effects of therapeutic creative dance. Revista Neurología. 2019;**68**:190-198

[74] Wu H-Y, Tsao T-H, Hsu C-H, Tu J-H, Yang C-B. The effects of low-impact dance on knee torque and lower extremity mobility in middle-aged and older women. Journal of Nursing Research. 2011;**19**(4):267-274

[75] Kim C-G, June K-J, Song R. Effects of a health-promotion program on cardiovascular risk factors, health behaviors, and life satisfaction in institutionalized elderly women. International Journal of Nursing Studies. 2003;**40**(4):375-381

[76] Kaltsatou A, Mameletzi D, Douka S. Physical and psychological benefits of a 24-week traditional dance program in breast cancer survivors. Journal of Bodywork and Movement Therapies. 2011;**15**(2):162-167

[77] Argiriadou E, Mountakis K, Konstantinakos P, Zakas A, Mavrovouniotis F, Mavrovounioti C. The effect of a single bout of greek dances on subjective health of middle-aged people. Journal of Physical Education and Sport. 2013;**13**(2):177-183

[78] Cernuda A. The arts in clinical health programs for the recovery of diseases and to improve quality of life. En B. Llamas, M. D. Storch, & L. F. Mazadiego (Eds.). Case Study of Innovative Projects - Successful Real Cases. London: IntechOpen; 2017. pp. 263-278. DOI: 10.5772/intechopen.69344)

[79] Cernuda A, de Andrés A. The benefits of Cuban psychoballet in the treatment of patients with Alzheimer´s disease. Psychometric validation. Revista de Información Científica. 2019;**98**(2):171-183

[80] Barnes J. Drama to promote social and personal well-being in six- and seven-year-olds with communication difficulties: The Speech Bubbles project. Perspectives in Public Health. 2014;**134**(2):101-109

[81] Anderson S, Fast J, Keating N, Eales J, Chivers S, Barnet D. Translating Knowledge: Promoting health through intergenerational community arts programming. Health Promotion Practice. 2017;**18**(1):15-25

[82] Wimpenny K, Savin-Baden M. Using Theatre and performance for promoting health and wellbeing amongst the 50+ community. The International Journal of Social, Political and Community Agendas in the Arts. 2014;**8**(1):47-64

[83] de Chumaceiro CLD. A Note on poetry therapy in health care training programs. Journal of Poetry Therapy Volume. 2000;**13**:219-223

[84] Xiang DH, Yi AM. A Look back and a path forward: Poetry's healing power during the pandemic. Journal of Medical Humanities. 2020;**41**(4):603-608

[85] Özsavran M. Mandala Art Therapy Mothers of Children wıth Special Needs Effect on Comfort Level: Randomızed Controlled Operatıon. Isparta: Zonguldak Bülent Ecevit University; 2022

Chapter 8

An Appropriate Quit Smoking Program for Thai People during the Covid-19 Pandemic

Thawalsak Ratanasiri, Chanchanok Aramrat, Somnuk Apiwantanagul, Bangonsri Jindawong, Thanawan Sirisuk and Amornrat Ratanasiri

Abstract

To find an appropriate quit smoking program on the spread of Covid-19 in Thailand during 2019–2021. To synthesize contents from Khon Kaen University (KKU) staffs' and students' research studies and projects from 1989 to 2021 about smoking problems and quit smoking programs and suggest appropriate quit smoking programs for Thai people during the Covid-19 pandemic. Fifteen publications and five projects presentation by the KKU staff and students were retrieved, reviewed, and analyzed. Smoking problems in Thai people were concerned. The Ministry of public health has disseminated knowledge of the dangers of smoking and has organization carried out all projects and campaigns of anti-smoking and had an anti-smoking act in the workplace on the Covid-19 pandemic during 2019–2021. Projects and research studies were able to help reduce these smoking problems. An appropriate quit smoking program needs to be developed and implemented. An appropriate quit smoking program needs to be implemented suitable for Thai people, in the hospitals, private clinics, families, and in the communities during the Covid-19 outbreak in Thailand.

Keywords: smoking problems, Covid-19 pandemic, appropriate quit smoking program, Thai people

1. Introduction

An appropriate quit smoking program is needed for Thai people because smoking is life-threatening and toxic to society. It affected others to be second-hand or third-hand smokers. So, it is a danger to the nation and people who get cigarette smoke from the public, in the workplaces, or in their houses. During the Coronavirus disease 2019 (Covid-19) outbreak, it was found that smokers who get diseases from smoking including cardiovascular diseases, chronic lung diseases, and diabetes are much more likely to be hospitalized or die if they catch coronavirus [1].

Covid-19 has triggered a global pandemic [2]. As of September 30th, 2021, 324 million cases had already been registered worldwide. The pandemic of Covid-19 has been very stressful, but there has never been a better time to quit smoking [3].

Quitting smoking is an important step to reduce the risk of developing cardiovascular complications. Smoking cigarettes makes the wall of the arteries sticky from the chemicals, so fatty material can stick to them. If the arteries that carry blood to the heart or brain get damaged and clogged, it leads to heart attack or stroke [4]. Smoking impairs lung function, making it harder for the body to fight off coronavirus and other diseases [5]. It is increasing the risk of severe illness, hospitalization, and death after being infected [3].

Smoking is different from other addictive drugs such as heroin, marijuana, and amphetamine, which have strict control by state and law and have a clear treatment. To protect people from smoking, the governments over the world only ask for operations and have a slogan, motivated to act and campaign to quit smoking since they found that smoking cigarette is an important cause of morbidity and mortality. Before the year 1981, there were 50,000 excess deaths per year in Britain, and 325,000 in the United States of America (USA) [6–8]. In Thailand, 10,000,000 Thai people were smokers in 1981, and at the time, most of them were teenagers [9]. The harms of tobacco use are well established, it causes 8 million deaths every year from cardiovascular diseases, respiratory diseases, cancers [10].

Since 2000, many countries chose the health of people instead of cigarettes: People in the USA had concerned of to be nonsmoking societies. The government of Canada had a smoking cessation program for the young generation. In Belgium, smoking had been prohibited in the public. Hong Kong and Singapore had created tobacco-free societies. India had prohibited smoking in close areas such as cinemas, on public transportations, in institutions, and in hospitals by law [11].

World Health Organization (WHO) has been concerned about smoking problems and set "the World No Tobacco Day." The first date was May 31, 1988, and has a slogan every year to persuade people to quit smoking. Most slogans since 1987 have encouraged people to be aware of their health and others' health. However, since 2020, the slogan needs people to quit smoking to avoid the severity of coronavirus infection. In 2020, it was "Addicted to Cigarettes, Addicted to Covid-19, High risk of Death# Quit Smoking, Reduce the Risk," and in 2021, it was "Quit Smoking, Reduce the Risk, You Can" [12].

This study aimed to find an appropriate quit smoking program for Thai people on the spread of Covid-19 in Thailand during 2019–2021.

2. Objectives

1. To synthesize contents from Khon Kaen University (KKU) staffs' and students' research studies and projects from 1989 to 2021 about smoking problems and quit smoking programs.

2. To find an appropriate quit smoking program for Thai people during the Covid-19 pandemic.

3. Methods

Fifteen publications and five project presentations by the KKU staff and students were retrieved, reviewed, and analyzed in two steps, to synthesize, and to find appropriate smoking programs.

The research review was approved by the Ethics Committee for Human Research at Khon Kaen University, Thailand (HE500637, HE513257, HE531310, HE551346, HE591188, Institutional Review Board Number (IRB 00001189), and Nepal Health Research Council (Reg. No 148/2021). Most of the research studies were based on secondary data. Those who volunteered had signed the consent form.

4. Results

There were two steps to these research results as follows:

In step 1: To synthesize contents from Khon Kaen University (KKU) staffs' and student's research studies and projects from 1989 to 2021 about smoking problems and quit smoking programs. It found that there were five groups of Thai people, for example, Thai males, Thai females, pregnant women, the youth and the students, and the workers, who need to quit smoking. Doctors who work in quit smoking clinics in hospitals or in private clinics can help them by treatment and counseling. Families and their communities can mentally support them as follows:

4.1 Synthesize contents of smoking problems

Research studies reported smoking problems presented; those Thai males smoke more than females in the universities [13–16] and in the factories [17–19]. Cigarette smoking was caused by substance abuse, for example, nicotine, tar, carbon monoxide, hydrogen cyanide, nitrogen dioxide, ammonia, formaldehyde, and cadmium [20]. Most of this substance abuse is caused by cancer and easily to be addicts [20]. Unfortunately, these reported that most of the smoking and drug addicts were the youth, 95.0% were males [19]. One hundred presented of drug addicts, 40.3% were unemployed, 15.5% were students [19]. Most of them got addicts as experimental (56.8%), harmful (24.2%), dependent (13.9%), and psychosis (5.1%) [19].

Smoking and substance abuse did people uncomfortable from chronic cough, tremor, and heart palpitation, no appetite, headache, moodiness, sleeplessness, wakefulness, and easy to get an accident, less of condom used risk to HIV/AIDS [21] and also were threatened by the law [18]. In the case of carbon monoxide (CO), measurement of breath CO level can be used in confirming smoking status, oral health, and factors related [22–25]. Some research reported that tobacco smoking is a risk indicator for periodontitis [26]. More dentists advised their patients to quit smoking [26].

The drug treatment system in Thailand has been classified into three types, namely the voluntary system, the correctional system, and the compulsory system. The compulsory system is under inhalant law and drug addict rehabilitation AC [27]. The research from the compulsory treatment system in Khon Kaen and Yasothon province about a relapse of methamphetamine users reported that 13 cases out of 65 cases were relapsed, and the left 52 cases were non-relapsed [17].

Researchers reported that family relationships and community participation can help children and youth from stressful and prohibit them from smoking or substance abuse. These research studies presented those children whose mothers look after them very closely had better growth development and better health than whose mothers worked outside the communities and left them to stay with their relatives [28]. In addition, it was found that marital status, occupational, and income were correlated in ascendant order to community participation in the youth's mental health [29].

4.2 Reviewed cases reported

Reviewed cases reported of quit smoking successful in each group of Thai people were as follows:

4.2.1 Thai male

One case reported that a Thai male who smoked since 1976 and was able to quit smoking in 2019 because of his health problem from an acute heart attack and need to insert three out of four catheters entering the heart. His doctor told him to stop smoking because it is a high risk of death from heart diseases and infected coronavirus. Before this, his parent and his family told him to stop smoking, because most of his family members are doctors. He cannot stop smoking, because he got stressed so easily. However, he prevented his family member from passive smoking when he smoked.

4.2.2 Thai female

One case reported a Thai female who smoked since she was very young, because of a broken family. She lived alone in the dormitory for study. During that time, she met her friends who have the same problems as her. Her friend persuaded her to smoke. She felt it made her comfortable and reduced her stress. She can quit smoking because she visited one beauty clinic, after she had a boyfriend, she found that her face looks older than other girls who were of the same age as her. Doctors in the beauty clinic told her that cigarette smoking made smokers look older than the others for 10 years. After she stops smoking, she looks younger and pretty. She was married and planned to have a baby, safe from passive smoking.

4.2.3 The pregnant woman

One case reported that it was very difficult for her to quit smoking because five people of her family member both males and females are smokers. They smoked in her house. She felt it was harder for her to quit smoking and avoid passive smoking. Because she loves her first baby very much, she can quit smoking by herself. But for the second and the third babies, she cannot stop smoking by herself, she needs to use candy and gum. However, she cannot stop smoking because her environment and the people around her are smokers. Finally, she quit smoking in 2010, after smoking since 2003 with helping from the Health Promotion Foundation (Thailand National Quitline: call 1600) [30].

4.2.4 The youth and one student

One case of the youth reported that he smoked and drank with his friends very often. He looked at his friend who smoked and drank, was very smart, and had the power over his group. One night he got into a motorcycle accident and needed to operate his dental and jaw. His parent felt so sad, he decided to quit smoking and drinking alcohol for his parent. In the case of one student, he smoked during his study in high school. He was able to stop smoking because he wants to be a good doctor and help the patient to quit smoking.

4.2.5 The worker

One case of a construction worker who smoked and drank every day since he was aged only 15 years old. His family asked him to stop smoking and drinking alcohol because he had one boy child aged 3 years old. His wife did not want his child to be passive smoking and feel that smoking and drinking are not good for his life. He cannot stop smoking and drinking until he was arrested and fined for drunk driving with serious penalties during the happy new year celebration for 2021. He can stop drinking, but smoking he cannot because his life was very stressful, smoking helped him to relax.

4.3 Reviewed five leading factors related

Reviewed five leading factors related to quitting smoking from five groups of Thai people. It prescribed that there are five leading factors as follows (see **Figure 1**).

a. Thai males' reasons for quitting smoking were (1) for their health, (2) to avoid diseases related to smoking and Covid-19 infected, (3) for their families, (4) for their friends, and (5) for their workplaces.

b. Thai females' reasons for quitting smoking were (1) for their self-image, (2) for their children and families, (3) for their health, (4) for their workplaces, and (5) to avoid diseases related to smoking and Covid-19 infected.

c. The pregnant women's reasons for quitting smoking were (1) for their babies, (2) for their self-image, (3) for their families, (4) for their friends, and (5) to avoid diseases related to smoking and Covid-19 infected.

d. The youths' reasons and the students' reasons for quitting smoking were (1) for their parent and their studies, (2) for their friends, (3) for their health, (4) to avoid diseases related to smoking and Covid-19 infected, and (5) for their societies.

e. The workers' reasons for quitting smoking were (1) for their health and employment, (2) for their workplaces, (3) for their employers, (4) to avoid diseases related to smoking and Covid-19 infected, and (5) for their families.

In step 2: To find an appropriate quit smoking program for Thai people during the Covid-19 pandemic: to develop an appropriate quit smoking program for each group of Thai people were three steps as follows (see **Figure 1**).

1. First step

    1.1 Reviewed research results about the smoking problems

    1.2 Concluded of factors related to smoking

    1.3 Reviewed of past cessation of quit smoking programs

2. Second step

2.1 History taking of bibliography, and smoking habits

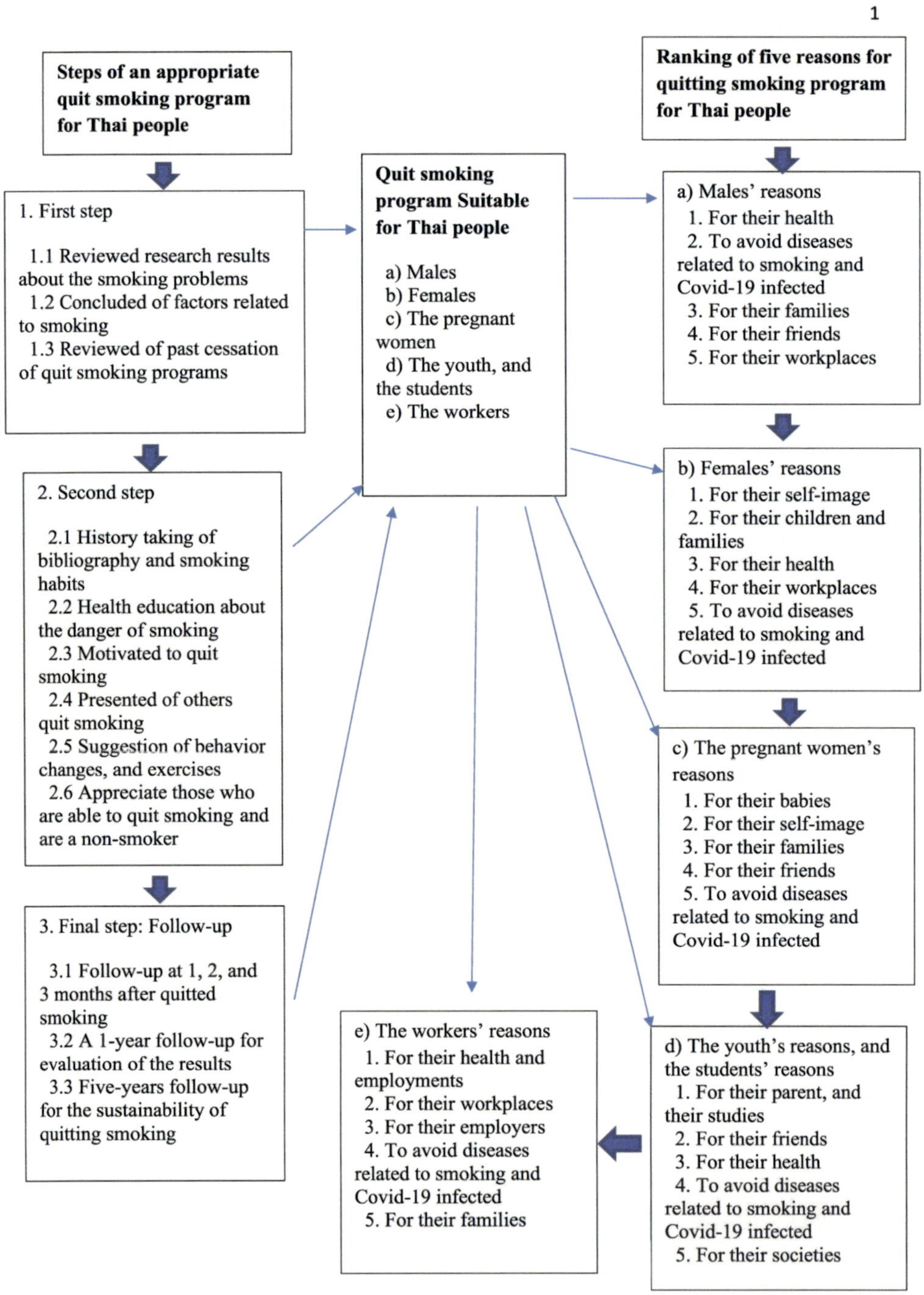

Figure 1.
An appropriate quit smoking program for Thai people in the year 2020–2021.

2.2 Health education about the dangers of smoking

2.3 Motivated to quit smoking

2.4 Presented of others quit smoking

2.5 Suggestion of behavior changes, and exercises

2.6 Appreciate those who are able to quit smoking and are a non-smoker.

3. Final step

3.1 Follow-up at 1, 2, and 3 months after quitted smoking

3.2 A 1-year follow-up for evaluation of the results

3.3 Five-years follow-up for the sustainability of quitting smoking

Appropriate Quit Smoking Program for Thai males, Thai females, the pregnant women, the youth and the students, and the workers need to the concerned of five reasons suitable for each group of Thai people, for example, the first leading related to quitting smoking for males was for their health, for females was for their self-image, for the pregnant women were for their babies, for the youth and the students were for their parents, and their studies, and for the workers were for their health and employment (see **Figure 1**).

In conclusion, smoking problems in Thai people were a concern. The Ministry of Public Health has discriminated knowledge regarding the dangers of smoking and has organization carry out all domeht and campaigns of anti-smoking and had Anti-Smoking Act, in the workplace on Covid-19 pandemic during 2019–2021. Projects and research studies were able to help reduce these smoking problems. An appropriate quit smoking program was developed and implemented to be suitable in each group during the Covid-19 pandemic as presented in **Figure 1**.

5. Discussions

From our study, it found that Thai males smoke more than Thai females, similar to Ji's report of the opposite idea of quitting smoking among Korean men and women, women smoked less than men and had a trend to quit smoking more than men [31]. Most of the smoking and drug addicts in Thailand were youth of 15 years old and older [9, 19]. They were unemployed (40.3%), and 15.5% were students [19]. The same as Karlan found that Filipinos aged 15 years or older were smokers up to 28.3%, and 22.5% smoked daily in 2009 [32]. About relapse of methamphetamine users in Northeast of Thailand reported that 13 cases out of 65 cases were relapsed, and the left 52 cases where non-relapse is closely reported of prior research with Filipinos that 72%, they wanted to stop smoking at some point, only 18% reported that they wanted to stop smoking now [32]. Our studies reported that family relationships and community participation can prohibit youth from smoking, similar to Garcia's report, which found that cessation programs for a smoking group should focus on changing the smokers' social environment and perception regarding the positive consequences of smoking in a way that is culturally sensitive and appropriate and considering the different levels of acculturation [33]. Complete prohibition of smoking in the household was one of the strongest correlates of successful quitting [33].

From our in-depth interview with women, one of them presented that she can quit smoking because she is concerned about her self-image. She found that her face looked older than her friends. She consulted doctors in a private clinic and desired to quit smoking. Similar to the government policy of the Philippines that persuades people to quit smoking for the self-image as "A Cigarette may out weight," results in the Philippines because some of them could quit smoking [32].

Our report of an appropriate quit smoking program for Thai people during the Covid-19 pandemic was reviewed from our research and our projects [34–38]. We are concerned about the individual differences for Thai males and females, the pregnant women, the youth and the students, and the workers. It found that the reasons for quitting smoking are in five leader reasons, but the difference in the first reason, most Thai males concerned of their health, Thai females concerned of their self-image, the pregnant women concerned of their babies, the youth and students concerned of their parents and their studies, and the workers concerned of their health and employment. Our quit smoking program had three steps, for example, first step, second step, and final step with 1, 2, and 3-month follow-up after quitting smoking, similar to the study of Nakhum District Hospital staffs [38] but in this study had another 1-year follow-up for evaluated the results of quitting, and 5-years follow-up for sustainable quit smoking. In our setting in the northeastern province such as Khon Kaen and Sakon Nakhon, they follow the Thai government policy and persuade people to quit smoking.

6. Conclusions

Smoking is an important problem in Thailand and over the world. It is a drug addict that causes severe diseases more than 200, such as lung cancer, chronic obstructive pulmonary disease (COPD), esophageal cancer, peptic cancer, gastrointestinal cancer, colon cancer, periodontitis, and asthma, it causes death from cancer.

Cigarette smoking and Covid-19 are complex interactions. During the pandemic, some reported that smokers are less likely to get the Coronavirus, while others reported smoking increased the risk of severe illness from it. A review by the World health Organization (WHO) found that smoking is associated with more severe illness and increased risk of death in people who need hospital treatment for Covid-19. Current smokers who get Coronavirus are twice as likely to attend hospital and tend to report more symptoms than non-smokers.

To control smoking, many countries had policies of Anti-Smoking Act, in the public, hospitals, institutions, in the families, in the communities, and in the workplaces. An appropriate quit smoking program needs to be developed and implemented, suitable for all Thai people in the hospitals, private clinics, families, and communities.

Strongest Thai government policies are of Anti-Smoking Act and control of Covid-19 pandemic. The physician and health personnel's role is to help patients to quit smoking and protect themselves from Coronavirus infection. Good family relationships participated from communities and societies with mental support can help reduce the problems of smoking, substance abuse, and also the Covid-19 pandemic.

Acknowledgements

The authors wish to thank (a) all the participants for their valuable contribution to this study, (b) provincial probation offices, the Department of Probation Office of the Narcotic Control Board, ISAN Substance Abuse Network, and Illicit Drugs Substance Abuse Academic Information Development Network for data support, and (c) Faculty of Dentistry and Faculty of Medicine, Khon Kaen University (KKU) for financial support.

Conflict of interest

All authors declare that they have no conflicts of interest.

Author details

Thawalsak Ratanasiri[1], Chanchanok Aramrat[2], Somnuk Apiwantanagul[3], Bangonsri Jindawong[4], Thanawan Sirisuk[5] and Amornrat Ratanasiri[6*]

1 Khon Kaen Hospital, Khon Kaen Province, Thailand

2 Faculty of Medicine, Department of Family Medicine, Chiang Mai University, Chiang Mai Province, Thailand

3 Sakon Nakhon Hospital, Sakon Nakhon Province, Thailand

4 Faculty of Medicine, Khon Kaen University, Khon Kaen Province, Thailand

5 Private Clinic in Bangkok, Bangkok, Thailand

6 Faculty of Medicine, Department of Community Medicine, Khon Kaen University, Khon Kaen Province, Thailand

*Address all correspondence to: amorat@kku.ac.th

References

[1] A UK Study Published in January 2021. Available from: https://thirax.bmj.com/content/early/2021/02/07/thoraxjnl-2020-216422 [Cited: 29 November 2021]

[2] Syed SA. Reviewed by Emily Henderson, COVID-19 and Smoking, News Medical Life Sciences. Available from: https://www.news-medical.net/health/COVID-19-andSmoking.aspx [Cited: 29 November 2021]

[3] Get Support to Quit Now. Available from: https://www.nhs.uk/better-health/quit-smoking/find-your-local-stop-smoking-service/ [Cited: 29 November 2021]

[4] Find Your Local Stop-Smoking Service. Available from: https://www.nhs.uk/smokefree/help-andadvice/local-support-services-helplines, or get support online and via Twitter at Today is the Day [Cited: 29 November 2021]

[5] World Health Organization. Smoking Impairs Lung Function Making It Harder for the Body to Fight Off Coronavirus and Other Diseases. Available from: https://www.who.int/news/item/11-05-2020-who-statement-tobacco-use-and-covid-19 [Cited: 29 November 2021]

[6] The Government of the Hong Kong Special Administrative Region. Census and Statistics Department, Hong Kong; 1976. In: Cheng KK, Lam TH, Ratanasiri A. Smoking among Medical Students in Hong Kong. Asia Pac J Public Health 1989;3(4):306-9. DOI:10.1177/101053958900300041

[7] The Government of the Hong Kong Special Administrative Region. Council on Smoking and Health, Hong Kong; 1976. In: Ratanasiri A, Cheng KK, Lam TH, Ratanasiri T. The Comparative Study about Medical Students' Knowledge and Attitude concerning Cigarette Smoking: A Study in Medical Students at Faculty of Medicine, Khon Kaen University, Khon Kaen, Thailand and at Faculty of Medicine, The University of Hong Kong, Hong Kong. Humanities and Social Sciences Journal 1992;10(1):111-7

[8] U.S. Department of Health, Education and Welfare Public Health Service. The Health Consequences of Smoking. Public Health Service Review; 1967. Public Health Service Publication No. 1696 [Revised: January 1968]

[9] National Statistics Offices. Surveyed Report Concerning Health and Social Welfare. Bangkok: National Statistics Offices, Thailand; 1981

[10] World Health Organization (WHO). Smoking and COVID-19. Scientific Brief. Available from: https://www.who.int/news-room/commentaries/detail/smoking-and-covid-19 [Cited: 29 November 2021]

[11] Mahler H. Between cigarettes and health; have to choose health. Thai Rural Doctor Club. 1928;**9**:8-10

[12] World Health Organization. WHO World No Tobacco Day. Available from: http://www.ashthailand.or.th/file.php?type=main-image&thumbnail=&file=612847-img-1335507896-1-3.jpg [Cited: 29 November 2021]

[13] Cheng KK, Lam TH, Ratanasiri A. Smoking among medical students in Hong Kong. Asia-Pacific Journal of Public Health. 1989;**3**(4):306-309. DOI: 10.1177/101053958900300041

[14] Ratanasiri A, Cheng KK, Ratanasiri T, Lam TH. Medical students' knowledge and attitude concerning cigarette smoking: A study in medical students at Faculty of Medicine, Khon Kaen University, Khon Kaen, Thailand. Srinagarind Medical Journal. 1992;**7**(1):17-27

[15] Ratanasiri A, Cheng KK, Lam TH, Ratanasiri T. The comparative study about medical students' knowledge and attitude concerning cigarette smoking: A study in medical students at Faculty of Medicine, Khon Kaen University, Khon Kaen, Thailand and at Faculty of Medicine, the University of Hong Kong, Hong Kong. Humanities and Social Sciences Journal. 1992;**10**(1):111-117

[16] NaNaKorn S, Osaka R, Chusilp K, Tsuda A, Maskasame S, Ratanasiri A. Gender differences in health-related practices among university students in Northeast Thailand. Asia-Pacific Journal of Public Health. 1999;**11**(1):10-15. DOI: 10.1177/101053959901100003

[17] Rodseeda P, Ratanasiri A, Kanato M, Pinitsoontorn S, Chiawiriyabunya I. An exploratory study on association between family relationship and relapse among methamphetamine users in compulsory treatment system of Khon Kaen and Yasothon Provinces. Journal of the Medical Association of Thailand. 2010;**93**(Suppl 3):S1-S5

[18] Jaichuang S, Ratanasiri A, Kanato M. Substance abuse among migrant workers of Thai-Laos Border, Thailand. Journal of the Medical Association of Thailand. 2012;**95**(9):1-6

[19] Watanaphithuk W, Ratanasiri A, Kanato M. Follow-up the outcome of treatment of inhalant users in Northeastern Thailand. Journal of the Medical Association of Thailand. 2013;**96**(7):854-859

[20] Likhitsathian S. Treatment for Quit Smoking. 24 December 2013. Available from: http://www.med.cmu.ac.th [Cited: 29 November 2021]

[21] Pant A, Kanato M, Ratanasiri A. Knowledge of and attitude towards HIV/AIDS and condom use among construction workers in the Kathmandu Valley Nepal. Journal of the Medical Association of Thailand. 2013;**96**:S107-S116

[22] Chatrchaiwiwatana S, Ratanasiri A. Exhhaled carbon monoxide level and smoking status in urban Khon Kaen adults. Journal of the Medical Association of Thailand. 2008;**91**(11):1669-1676

[23] Chatrchaiwiwatana S, Ratanasiri A. Exhaled carbon monoxide levels among tobacco smokers by age. The Southeast Asian Journal of Tropical Medicine and Public Health. 2017;**48**(2):429-437

[24] Chatrchaiwiwatana S, Ratanasiri A. Determination of smoking status among Thai employees by the best exhaled carbon monoxide cut-off level and association with oral health conditions. The Southeast Asian Journal of Tropical Medicine and Public Health. 2018;**49**(1):165-174

[25] Chatrchaiwiwatana S, Ratanasiri A. Association between exhaled carbon monoxide and oral health status in active and passive smokers. Journal of the Medical Association of Thailand. 2011;**94**(5):601-609

[26] Chatrchaiwiwatana S, Ratanasiri A. Periodontitis associated with tobacco smoking among rural Khon Kaen Thai males: Analysis of two data sets. Journal of the Medical Association of Thailand. 2009;**92**(1):1524-1531

[27] Probation Department, Ministry of Justice. Drug Addict Rehabilitation Act AD 2002. Ministry of Justice: Bangkok; 2008

[28] Leungtongkum P, Piniwatsoontorn S, Somnasang P, Kanato M, Ratanasiri A, Maskasame S, et al. Study groups of mother or relatives whose level of education are higher than prathom 4 which normally look after children better than the similar groups who have prathom 4 education or lower; and study different factors which influence the growth of preschool children. Srinagarind Hospital Medical Journal. 1987;**2**(1):23-29

[29] Ratanasiri A, Klomjit C, Methapat C. Community participation about the youth mental health. Srinagarind Hospital Medical Journal. 1989;**4**(2):121-129

[30] Doungtong T. Quit Smoking for Children, it is the Duty of the Word Mother [online]. Available from: http://20th.thaihealth.or.th [Accessed: 30 June 2017]

[31] Ji M, Hofstetter CR, Hovell M, Irvin V, Song YJ, Lee J, et al. Smoking cessation patterns and predictors among adult Californians of Korean descent. Nicotine & Tobacco Research. 2005;**7**(1):59-69. DOI: 10.1080/14622200412331328493

[32] Karlan D, Zinman J, Giné X. CARES Commitment Savings for Smoking Cessation in the Philippines. Available from: https://www.povertyactionlab.org/evaluation/cares-commitment-savings-smoking-cessation-philippines [Cited: 29 November 2021]

[33] Garcia GM, Romero RA, Maxwell AE. Correlates of smoking cessation among Filipino immigrant men. Journal of Immigrant and Minority Health. 2010;**12**(2):259-262. DOI: 10.1007/s10903-009-9244-9

[34] Ratanasiri T, et al. Alcohol Abuse Project. East Asian Medical Students' Conference (EAMSC) 2011, Thailand [Accessed: 19-23 January 2011]

[35] Chaiear N, Paileeklee S, Jindawong B, Yimtae K, Thanawiratananij P, Thinkamrop B, et al. Smoking & worker health status in Khon Kaen Province 2002-2003. In: Poster Presentation on 5th Annual Conference of the International Society for the Prevention of Tobacco Induced Diseases at the University of Hong Kong, Hong Kong; 24-28 November 2006

[36] Sopontammarak A. Sakon Nakhon Model, No Smoking Campaign Model [online]. Available from: http://20th.thaihealth.or.th [Accessed: 9 March 2016]

[37] Apasakul S. Sakon Nakhon Pilot Project: Invites People in the Area to Quit Smoking [online]. Available from: http://20th.thaihealth.or.th [Accessed: 6 November 2019]

[38] Nakhum District Hospital. A study of smoking cessation model in village health volunteer at Nakhum Health Promotion Hospital, Huay Yang Subdistrict, Muang District, Sakon Nakhon Province. Available from: http://cupsakol.org/pkp2/pkp2/Sat24557.pdf [Cited: 29 November 2021]

Chapter 9

Perspective Chapter: Tobacco Control in Sub-Saharan Africa – Challenges and Recommendations

Aishat Jumoke Alaran, Fahd Adebola Khalid-Salako, Yusuff Adebisi Adebayo, Abubakar Olaitan Badmos, Oluwaseyifunmi Oladipo, Zainab Oluwatosin Onibon and Don Eliseo Lucero-Prisno III

Abstract

According to the World Health Organization, more than 80% of the world's current smokers live in low- and middle- income countries. In Sub-Saharan Africa (SSA), the increase in tobacco smoking is facilitated by the fast-growing population, increase in purchasing power of the consumers and massive efforts by the tobacco industry to expand their reach in this region. Until the World Health Organization's Framework Convention on Tobacco Control (FCTC), many countries in SSA had weak or non-existent tobacco control policies, about 44 countries in the region are currently signatories to the treaty. Despite being signatories to the FCTC, many sub-Saharan African countries have not been able to implement and/or enforce comprehensive tobacco control policies. This chapter is intended to share the challenges facing existing public health advocacy and interventions against tobacco smoking in SSA countries and to make recommendations necessary to control tobacco smoking in the SSA countries.

Keywords: tobacco control, sub-Saharan Africa, smoking, FCTC, harm reduction

1. Introduction

Tobacco use poses a major threat to global public health [1]. The number of smokers globally has now risen to 1.3 billion and may reach 1.5 billion by 2025 with low-and-middle-income countries (LMICs) having 80% of the global smoking population [2, 3]. By 2025, the smoking rate in sub-Saharan Africa is estimated to be about 37%, the highest estimated growth among the six World Health Organization (WHO) regions [4].

African countries are therefore positioned on the upward slope of the smoking prevalence curve, denoting a high vulnerability to further penetration of markets by multinational tobacco corporations through advertising, increased competition for sales and large-scale promotion of appealing images of smokers, encouraging experimental smoking [5–7]. Effective tobacco control is imperative in Africa as it is well-documented in literature that the region is suffering from the double burden of communicable and non-communicable diseases [8].

The answer to the increasing danger of the global tobacco epidemic is often pointed to as the WHO Framework Convention on Tobacco Control (FCTC) by the anti-tobacco advocacy groups, which is the first international treaty on tobacco control [9]. MPOWER is another policy package intended to aid in the country-level implementation of effective interventions to reduce the demand for tobacco, as ratified by WHO FCTC. The six evidence-based components of MPOWER are: Monitor tobacco use and prevention policies; Protect people from tobacco smoke; Offer help to quit tobacco use; Warn about the dangers of tobacco; Enforce bans on tobacco advertising, promotion and sponsorship; Raise taxes on tobacco [10].

Looking at the status of legislation on tobacco control in Africa, Sub-Saharan Africa (SSA) countries are still far from the benchmark on implementation of the FCTC stipulations. In countries like South Africa and Kenya, favorable political environments and adequate knowledge provide fertile grounds for the implementation of FCTC and the MPOWER measures while in countries like Nigeria, Malawi and Ghana, prioritization, lack of enforcement of existing tobacco control initiatives, and lack of capacity are factors shown to be major obstacles hindering effective policy implementation [7, 11–13].

Many advocacy groups and governments use the MPOWER policy package and the WHO FCTC as the benchmark for tobacco-related advocacy. To ensure the success of FCTC, a formal agreement of the ratification must be followed by implementation tailored to the particular challenges of SSA countries, putting to use, lessons from schemes that have been proven to work in other environments. There is emerging advocacy for Tobacco Harm Reduction, an option proven to reduce the harm from tobacco consumption with alternative nicotine products such as e-cigarettes and snus, in SSA by some advocacy groups.

2. Case

Many African countries are struggling to implement the recommendations of the treaty in a way that matches the unified action of member countries during the treaty negotiations. Implementation of the FCTC recommendations varies greatly across the SSA countries ranging from 9% in Sierra Leone to 78% in Kenya [14].

South Africa is making strides in tobacco control, putting to use a couple of opportunities presented by the African National Congress [12]. It has successfully put in place, legislation that bans smoking in outdoor locations and has introduced bans on smoking in other public places. It became the first country in the world to have a national ban on smoking in cars where children (≤12 years) are present and also made significant efforts towards a smoke-free world cup in 2010 [12].

Nigeria's first attempt to control tobacco consumption in furtherance of public health was in the form of the Tobacco (Control) decree in 1990 [12]. A National Tobacco Control Act (NTCA), 2015 was signed into law after the presidency had earlier refused to assent to an earlier Tobacco Control bill that was passed in the senate and house of representatives in 2011 [13]. The NTCA as it is, contains significant loopholes that loosen its ultimate control over the production, sale, and distribution of tobacco in the country.

A National Tobacco Control Committee (NATOCC) was created to advise the Federal Ministry of Health (FMoH) on the implementation of tobacco control policies. The NATOCC however, includes representatives of the Manufacturers Association of Nigeria (MAN) (which includes the tobacco industry), in violation of Article 5.3 of the WHO FCTC, providing an avenue for the tobacco industry to influence the implementation of the tobacco control policies [13]. The act also requires that regulations proposed by the Federal Ministry of Health (FMoH) be approved by both houses of the National Assembly, reducing the independence of the FMoH and allowing the industry ample opportunity to influence tobacco control by lobbying with legislators. The Standards Organization of Nigeria (SON), developed the Nigerian Industrial Standards (NIS) for cigarettes, responsible for the control of the constituents and emissions of cigarettes, and with the backing of the laws governing the organization, involved the tobacco industry and excluded the FMoH in the development of the NIS [13].

Kenya passed its first tobacco Control Bill in 1998 and made history by being the second country in the world to ratify and sign the WHO FCTC on the same day in 2014. Kenya also passed its first post-FCTC control bill in 2007 [12]. Strong local evidence on the economic effects of tobacco use, coupled with political factors provided the required impetus for the development and implementation of strategies by Kenya to control the production, sale, and distribution of tobacco in Kenya. The Tobacco Control Act (TCA)←←←← of 2007 developed to implement the WHO FCTC policies remains the main tobacco control policy document in Kenya. The provisions of the TCA have been implemented in Kenya although there is room for improvement [7]. The Finance Act in Kenya has stipulated an increase in the excise duty of tobacco products at 35% (which however remains lower than the 70% recommended by the WHO) [7]. Tobacco smoking has now been banned in all public places with enforcement in most areas. Although, signs and billboards can still be found in certain parts of the country [15], advertisement, promotion, and sponsorship has been completely banned in the country by the TCA [12].

Malawi, despite having five documents on tobacco and tobacco smoking is not a signatory to WHO FCTC [12]. Besides this, the Malawian economy is largely reliant on tobacco farming and implementation of some articles of the WHO FCTC according to key players, is feared by the government and has received resistance from farmers and the tobacco industry [12]. With the belief that ratifying parts of the FCTC to limit exposure to tobacco smoke will lead to the implementation of all aspects of the FCTC, including Articles 17 and 18, which discourage support for tobacco farming and will have an untoward impact on the national economy due to their reliance on tobacco farming as their cash crop in Malawi [12, 16]. Foundation for Smoke-free World has been working with national authorities, partners, and tobacco farmers to help smallholder tobacco farmers transit to alternative livelihoods.

A paradoxical observation made during the study of the global rate of reduction in tobacco smoking to observe changes in the rate after 2003 was that while there was no significant difference in the rates of reduction of tobacco smoking -before and after 2003- globally, stratified analyses showed that European and other high income countries have seen increased rates of reductions in tobacco smoking while low-and-middle-income countries and Asian countries have seen a reversal in the reducing rate of tobacco smoking after the adoption of FCTC in 2003 in such a way that LMICs as well as Asian countries are consuming in excess of what they used to, enough cigarettes to make up for the reduction in consumption in their high income and European counterparts [17]. A possible explanation would be that implementation of FCTC provisions in high income and European countries have facilitated the shift in focus of the tobacco industry to LMICs and Asian countries where governmental control is not as stringent [9].

Therefore, the role the tobacco industry plays in the effectiveness of FCTC in SSA countries cannot be overestimated. Ranging from allegedly sponsoring "researches" and analyses that debunk the WHO claims about the health hazards of tobacco smoking, to mongering the notion among stakeholders in SSA countries that relates reduction in tobacco cultivation with malignant economic trends, the tobacco industry is indeed clawing back at the initiatives put forward to curb tobacco smoking in the grand stages of policy making and nuances of implementation.

In complement with the FCTC, Tobacco Harm Reduction (THR) provides another option worth exploring. It involves the use of less harmful nicotine products, e.g., snus and e-cigarettes as a substitute for tobacco smoking. Many tobacco control advocacy groups such as the Nigeria Tobacco Control Alliance, the Environmental Rights Action/Friends of the Earth Nigeria and Campaign for Tobacco-Free Kids among others strongly resist the concept of THR because of misconceptions surrounding the use of these products, e.g., exaggerated health impacts of nicotine and normalization of the use of these products among others.

Nonetheless, the use of these products is increasing globally and SSA will not be an exception. Additionally, there is an increase in a number of tobacco harm reduction advocacy groups in SSA, e.g., Tobacco Harm Reduction Nigeria, Tobacco Harm Reduction Kenya, Tobacco Harm Reduction Malawi, Tobacco Harm Reduction Uganda and Campaign for Safer Alternatives among others. Moreover, the first tobacco harm reduction forum by Campaign for Safer Alternatives is scheduled to hold in Nairobi, Kenya but was canceled because of the unprecedented novel coronavirus pandemic.

3. Discussion

Being a pacesetter, the FCTC was undoubtedly a much-needed stride in the control of the global tobacco epidemic. However, it requires adaptation to overcome the significant challenges it faces in the developing world. It is, therefore, necessary to incorporate some concepts not covered in FCTC and MPOWER if the public health implications of tobacco smoking in SSA are to be checked.

The status quo dictates that current smokers have only two options, complete cessation and abstinence from tobacco or continued use in the face of overwhelming evidence of the harmful effects of tobacco smoking on the health of the user, bystanders, and on the environment [18, 19]. A lot of smokers are unable, or unwilling to stop smoking, and the majority of those who quit, relapse within months. This necessitates the introduction of a third option that caters for those that are unable to quit smoking while producing less harm than that produced from traditional tobacco smoking; Tobacco Harm Reduction [18].

Despite being relatively new in SSA, the concept of THR is not new in the western part of the world, having had its fair share of controversies and debates. It has also proven efficacious in the reduction of the prevalence of tobacco smoking as observed in Sweden and Norway with the THR product, Snus [18, 20]. A THR product that is garnering support is the e-cigarette which due to its appearance and mode of use, is touted to imitate the social cues of smoking traditional cigarettes and therefore, provide better help with components of addiction to tobacco smoking not directly related to the addictive component, nicotine.

There is not enough evidence to prove that THR products are absolutely safe when used as intended as e-cigarette vapor for instance contain potentially toxic compounds [18, 19] . However, they are much safer alternatives, devoid of the contaminants and toxic combustion products of cigarettes. They have toxicity profiles, comparable with the FDA-approved pharmaceutically-formulated smoking-cessation aids [18]. THR advocacy groups continue to advocate the inclusion of "ED" to MPOWER policy package so it can become MPOWERED, where E is Encourage Safer Alternatives and D is Deliver accurate & honest information regarding THR.

Successful reduction of the public health risk of tobacco smoking in SSA will require that policymakers at all levels deploy schemes and policies that allow for better acceptance and market flow of THR products while keeping stringent measures on tobacco smoking. Extensive research will also be required to keep tabs on the socio-economic effects of substituting THR products for traditional cigarettes, as well as on public health and the prevailing perspective and practice of healthcare providers.

Funding information

The authors receive no financial support for the research and authorship of this article.

Conflict of interest

Aishat Jumoke Alaran and Yusuff Adebayo Adebisi are both beneficiaries of the Tobacco Harm Reduction Scholarship Programme by Knowledge-Action-Change, London. Aishat Jumoke Alaran is a 2020 beneficiary while Yusuff Adebayo Adebisi is a 2019 beneficiary. Both authors are advocates of Tobacco Harm Reduction.

Author details

Aishat Jumoke Alaran[1,2*], Fahd Adebola Khalid-Salako[1,2], Yusuff Adebisi Adebayo[3,4], Abubakar Olaitan Badmos[5], Oluwaseyifunmi Oladipo[3], Zainab Oluwatosin Onibon[2] and Don Eliseo Lucero-Prisno III [4,6]

1 National Institute for Pharmaceutical Research and Development, Abuja, Nigeria

2 Faculty of Pharmaceutical Sciences, University of Ilorin, Ilorin, Nigeria

3 Faculty of Public Health, Department of Human Nutrition and Dietetics, University of Ibadan, Ibadan, Nigeria

4 Global Health Focus, London, United Kingdom

5 National Primary Healthcare Development Agency, Abuja, Nigeria

6 Department of Global Health and Development, London School of Hygiene and Tropical Medicine, London, United Kingdom

*Address all correspondence to: alaranaishat@gmail.com

References

[1] Alfred L, Jnr D, Fabyan M, Dei LA Jr. The threats of globalization on global public health with specific reference to tobacco control. Public Health Research. 2016;**6**:132

[2] World Heath Organization. Global action plan for the prevention and control of noncommunicable diseases. Geneva Switzerland: World Health Organization 2013-2020; 2013

[3] Jha P, Peto R. Global effects of smoking, of quitting, and of taxing tobacco. The New England Journal of Medicine. 2014;**370**:60

[4] Bilano V, Gilmour S, Moffiet T, D'Espaignet ET, Stevens GA, Commar A, et al. Global trends and projections for tobacco use, 1990-2025: An analysis of smoking indicators from the WHO Comprehensive information Systems for Tobacco Control. Lancet. 2015;**385**:966-976

[5] Pampel F. Tobacco use in sub-Sahara Africa: Estimates from the demographic health surveys. Social Science & Medicine. 2008;**66**:1772

[6] Siddiqi K. Tobacco use in sub-Saharan Africa: The risks and challenges. Nicotine & Tobacco Research. Oxford University Press. 2019;**21**:999

[7] Magitta NF. Epidemiology of tobacco use and dependence in Sub-Saharan Africa: A systematic review. Journal of Pulmonology and Clinical Research. 2018;**2**(1):9-15

[8] Lucero-Prisno DE, Adebisi YA, Lin X. Current efforts and challenges facing responses to 2019-NCoV in Africa. Global Health Research and Policy. 2020;**5**:21

[9] Hoffman SJ, Poirier MJP, Rogers Van Katwyk S, Baral P, Sritharan L. Impact of the WHO framework convention on tobacco control on global cigarette consumption: Quasi-experimental evaluations using interrupted time series analysis and in-sample forecast event modelling. British Medical Journal. 2019;**365**:1

[10] World Heath Organization. WHO Report on the Global Tobacco Epidemic 2019. Offer Help to Quit Tobacco Use; 2019

[11] Owusu-Dabo E, McNeill A, Lewis S, Gilmore A, Britton J. Status of implementation of framework convention on tobacco control (FCTC) in Ghana: A qualitative study. BMC Public Health. 2010;**10**:1

[12] Wisdom JP, Juma P, Mwagomba B, Ndinda C, Mapa-Tassou C, Assah F, et al. Influence of the WHO framework convention on tobacco control on tobacco legislation and policies in sub-Saharan Africa. BMC Public Health. 2018;**18**:954-965

[13] Egbe CO, Bialous SA, Glantz S. Framework convention on tobacco control implementation in Nigeria: Lessons for low- a Nd middle-income countries. Nicotine & Tobacco Research. 2019;**21**:1122

[14] Brathwaite R, Addo J, Smeeth L, Lock K. A systematic review of tobacco smoking prevalence and description of tobacco control strategies in sub-Saharan African countries; 2007 to 2014. 2015;**1**

[15] Shoba J. Best practices in implementation of article 13 of the WHO FCTC case study: Kenya, 2013. 2013;**13**

[16] Otañez MG, Mamudu HM, Glantz SA. Tobacco companies' use of developing countries' economic reliance on tobacco to lobby against global tobacco control: The case of Malawi. American Journal of Public Health. 2009;**99**:1759

[17] Eriksen M, Mackay J, Ross H. The Tobacco Atlas. 4th ed. Atlanta, GA: World Lung Foundation. Available from: http://Tobaccoatlas.Org/; World Med. Heal. Policy 5, 2742013

[18] Polosa R, Rodu B, Caponnetto P, Maglia M, Raciti C. A fresh look at tobacco harm reduction: The case for the electronic cigarette. Harm Reduction Journal. 2013;**10**:1

[19] Nansseu JRN, Bigna JJR. Electronic cigarettes for curbing the tobacco-induced burden of noncommunicable diseases: Evidence revisited with emphasis on challenges in sub-Saharan Africa. Pulmonary Medicine. 2016;**2016**

[20] Ramström L, Borland R, Wikmans T. Patterns of smoking and SNUS use in Sweden: Implications for public health. International Journal of Environmental Research and Public Health. 2016;**13**:1

Chapter 10

Tobacco Use in Bangladesh

Papia Sultana

Abstract

Bangladesh is rich in cultural inheritance and tobacco use is an integral part of the culture in the country. Bangladesh is a tobacco-producing country and one of the most consuming countries. Traditionally, Bangladeshi male tobacco users mostly smoke cigarettes and *bidi*, and chew tobacco leaves such as *zarda, sadapata, gul, and khaini*. However, females usually do not smoke tobacco but chew tobacco leaves. According to Global Adult Tobacco Survey (GATS) Bangladesh, 2017, 40.0% of males and 25.2% of females use tobacco; among them, 36.2% of males and 0.8% of females smoked cigarettes or other forms of smoking tobacco such as *bidi* or *hukkah*; and 16.2% of males and 24.8% of females use smokeless tobacco (betel quid with *zarda, gul, sadapata*, etc.). This chapter has presented a description of tobacco use and its socio-demographic and economic correlates, secondhand tobacco exposure, tobacco use policies in workplaces and residences, awareness, quitting methods, and management of marketing and media coverage in Bangladesh.

Keywords: tobacco use, secondhand smoking, smokeless tobacco, e-cigarette, quitting method, media and marketing of tobacco, Bangladesh

1. Introduction

Bangladesh has a rich cultural inheritance. Tobacco use is an integral part of the culture in the country. Bangladesh has an extended history of tobacco use and, smoked and smokeless tobacco is used in different ways. Bangladesh is also a tobacco-producing country. About 46,472 hectares of land is used for cultivating tobacco and about 87,628 tons of tobacco leaf is produced every year [1]. Bangladesh stands at 14th position in area under tobacco production, 12th position for production in quantity, and contributes 1.3% of global tobacco production [1]. Usually, males in Bangladesh smoke cigarettes and *bidi*, and use raw or formatted tobacco leaves such as *zarda, sadapata, gul, khoinee*, etc. Although tobacco smoking among females is not well accepted in the country, chewing tobacco leaf is acceptable. Tobacco-related death and illness hamper the social and economic progression of a country. Early death or disability from tobacco use decreases the living standards and obstructs the financial condition of the family [2]. A prospective study of ten years with twenty thousand adult participants in Bangladesh has discovered that smoking was accountable for 25% of male deaths and 7.6% of female deaths directly or indirectly [3], which clearly visualize that Bangladesh has experienced a large number of tobacco-related deaths and illnesses that authorized national as well as global attention to this massive delinquent. It is also estimated that about 1.2 million people became ill due to tobacco use. The economic cost of tobacco is enormous, which is about 863 million USD each year [4].

Recently Bangladesh has been going through health and economic evolution, and has experienced a dual burden of communicable and noncommunicable diseases. Tobacco is identified as the key risk factor for noncommunicable diseases. Deaths due to tobacco are projected to be declined by 9% from 2002 to 2030 in developed countries, but increased to double in low- and middle-income countries. Like many other countries, the Government of Bangladesh has executed some steps to minimize tobacco use. Recently, the National Strategic Plan of Action for Tobacco Control (2007-2010) has been executed in the country. The MPOWER package is a series of six recognized strategies, which had been launched in Bangladesh in December 2008. But, Government has failed to make the acts 100% in action. On the other hand, teenagers are getting more prevalent to tobacco use. Smoking affects adversely the individual smoker, in some cases his/her family and society as a whole. A significant amount of costs is being used for medicinal purposes, leaving the family in poorer economic condition. It also reduces the individuals' working capacity. All these are alarming to Bangladesh.

This chapter will provide a detailed description of tobacco use and its socio-demographic and economic correlates, secondhand tobacco exposure, tobacco use policies in workplaces and residences, awareness, quitting methods, and management of marketing and media coverage in Bangladesh.

2. Tobacco use and its correlates

Tobacco is used in various forms and patterns in Bangladesh. There are different types of tobacco, e.g., smoked tobacco and smokeless tobacco. Main tobacco smoking products are manufactured cigarettes and *bidi*. Water pipe (hookah), pipe, cigars, e-cigarettes, shisha, hand-rolled cigarettes, etc. are also available. Global Adult Tobacco Survey (GATS) Bangladesh 2017 reported that overall 18.0% (19.2 million) adults currently smoke some form of tobacco, with 36.2% men and 0.8% women [5]. Among the smokers, 77.1% smokes manufactured cigarettes, 29.0% smokes *bidis*, 0.5% smokes water pipe (hookah), 0.4% smokes hand-rolled cigarette, 0.3% smokes cigar, cheroot, or cigarillo, 0.2% smokes tobacco in pipe, and 0.2% smokes tobacco in other way (**Figure 1**). Various studies have reported that tobacco smoking is associated with male gender, middle age, low education, low paid jobs and lower economic condition [6]. However, some studies also identified that peer smoking, higher grades in academic results, higher amount of pocket money, etc. are positively associated with tobacco smoking in teenagers [7].

There are many types of smokeless tobacco (SLT) products that have traditionally been used in Bangladesh. Smokeless tobacco ranges from unprocessed to processed with various attractive flavors and forms including *Zarda, Gul, Sada Pata, Pan Masala, and Khaini* (**Figure 2**).

Zarda is the most common smokeless tobacco product used in Bangladesh. It is a processed tobacco leaf. Usually, tobacco leaf is boiled, baked, or roasted and flaked. The flakes of tobacco leaf are then mixed with other spices, sweeteners, and flavors, especially menthol and camphor, herbs, fragrances, saffron, and silver flakes (**Figure 3**). It is usually used with betel quid with slaked lime paste and chopped areca nut (**Figure 4**), and is very popular among older men and women.

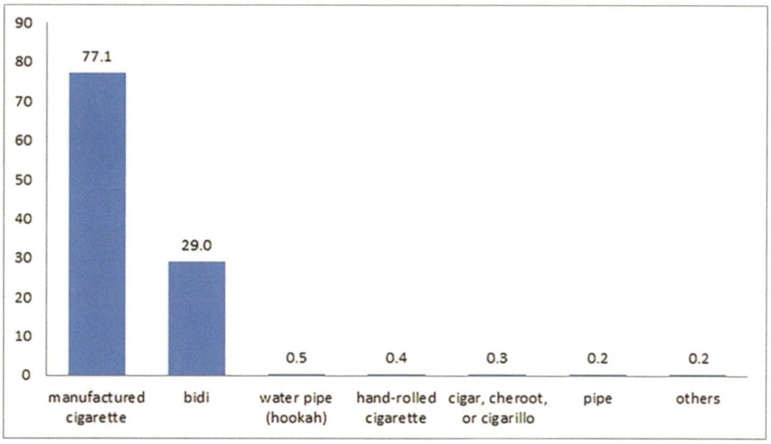

Figure 1.
Prevalence of tobacco smoking in Bangladesh, GATS 2017.

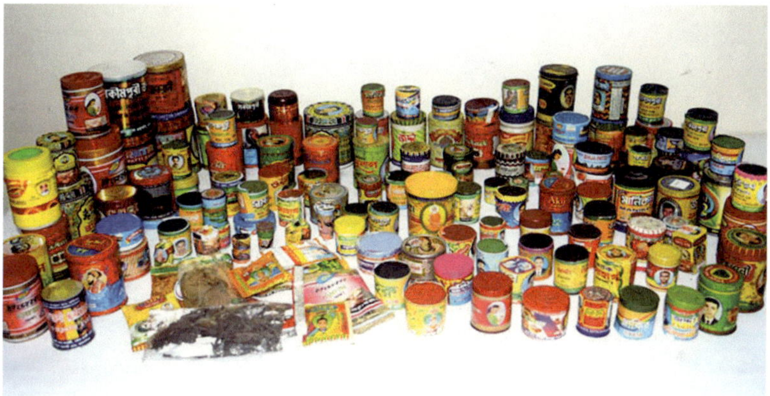

Figure 2.
Smokeless tobacco products in Bangladesh.

Gul is the powdered tobacco product with the ash of tendu leaves, usually sold in small containers or sachets (**Figure 5**). It is used to clean teeth, but sometimes it is placed in mouth between the gums and lips for few minutes before cleaning teeth.

Sada Pata is the raw tobacco leaf (**Figure 6**), which is dried and is usually used for chewing among low-socioeconomic people.

PanMasala with tobacco (PM-T) is a mixture of crushed tobacco leaf, chopped areca nut, lime, catechu, and spices (**Figure 7**). It is used in betel leaf and is very popular among teenagers due to its nice flavor.

Khaini is made from crushed sun-dried tobacco leaves (**Figure 8**). A small amount of crushed and fermented tobacco is taken in the palm and a pinch of slaked lime paste is added to it. The mixture becomes ready to use after it is rubbed thoroughly with the thumb. Traditionally, a user prepares this at the time of use. It is put in the mouth and sucked or chewed slowly. Users may add areca nut if they like. Usually, a special group of people in Bangladesh use *Khaini*.

According to GATS Bangladesh 2017, overall 20.6% of adults use smokeless tobacco products with 16.2% males and 24.8% females. Among the smokeless tobacco users, 71.8% use Betel leaf with zarda, only zarda, or zarda with superi, 28.0% use Betel

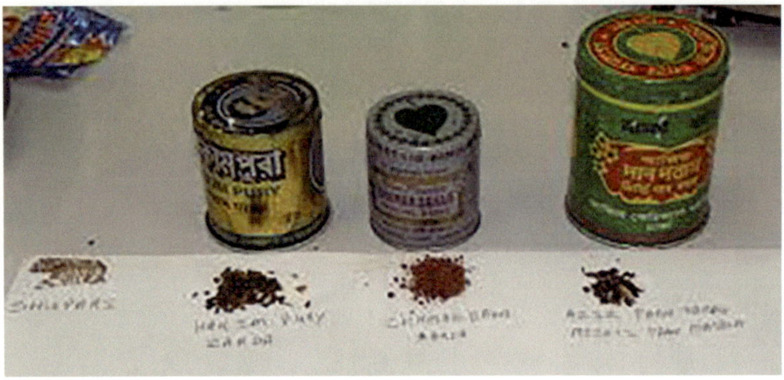

Figure 3.
Zarda.

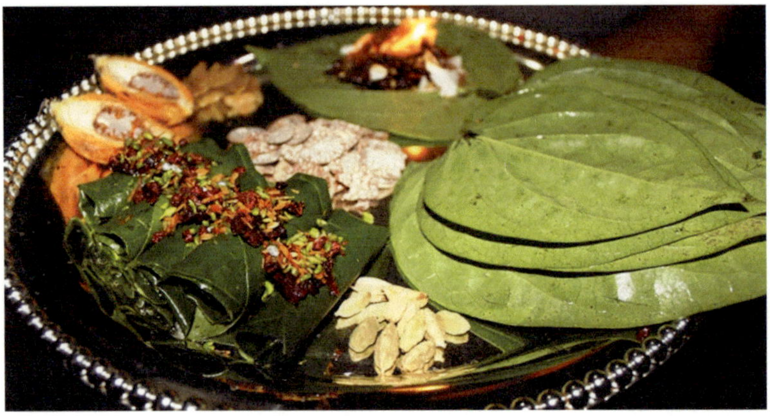

Figure 4.
Betel quid with Zarda.

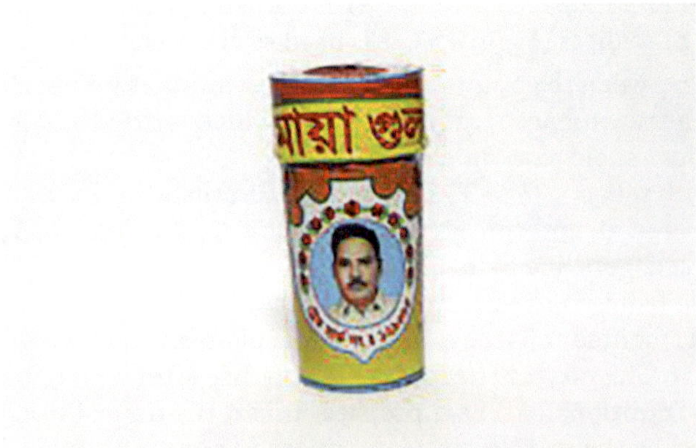

Figure 5.
Gul.

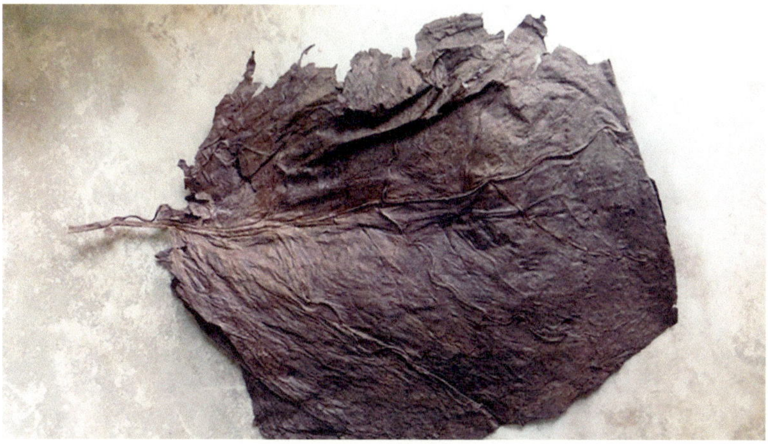

Figure 6.
Sada Pata.

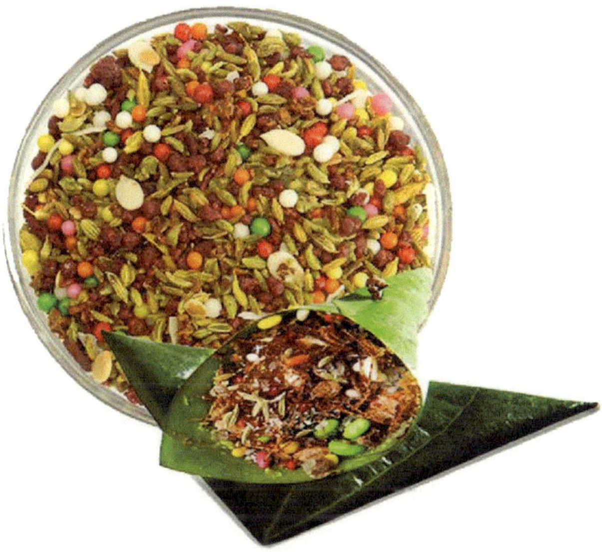

Figure 7.
PanMasala.

leaf with Sada Pata, 8.1% use Gul, 3.6% use Pan Masala with tobacco, 2.3% chew only Sada Pata, 0.7% use Khaini, and 0.2% use smokeless tobacco products in other forms (**Figure 9**). Smokeless tobacco use is associated with the female gender, middle age and older people, and people with low education, low-paid jobs, and low economic conditions.

E-cigarettes (electronic-cigarettes) [8, 9] are still fairly new in Bangladesh. E-cigarette is an electronic device that mimics tobacco smoking. E-cigarettes are available in many shapes and sizes in Bangladesh (**Figure 10**). Common structure of the device is to have a battery, a heating component, and a chamber to hold a liquid

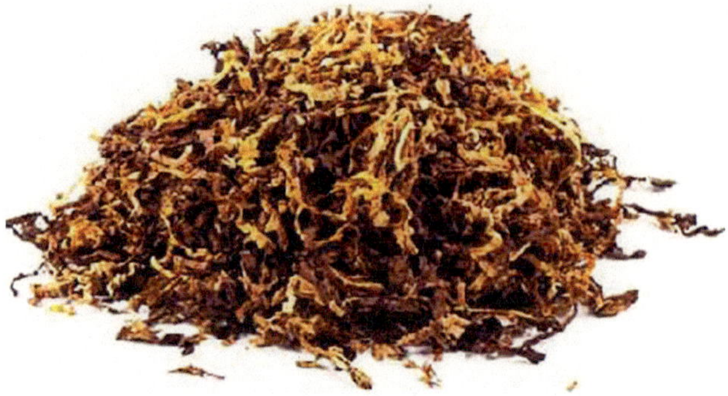

Figure 8.
Khaini.

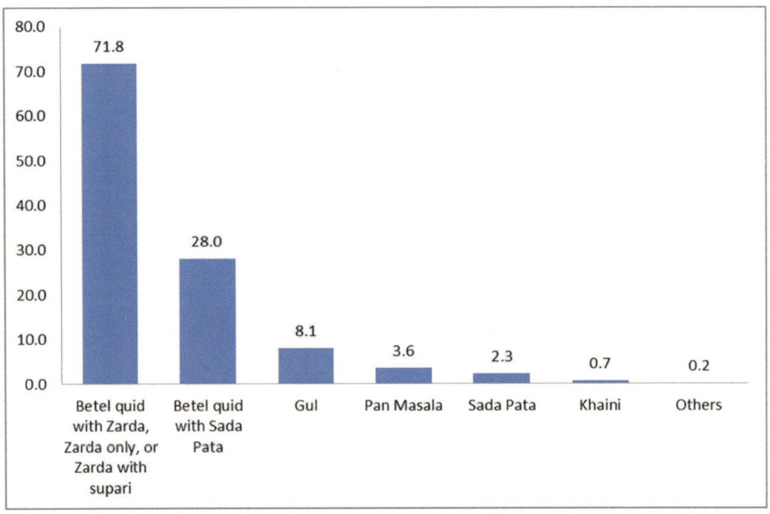

Figure 9.
Prevalence of smokeless tobacco use in Bangladesh, GATS 2017.

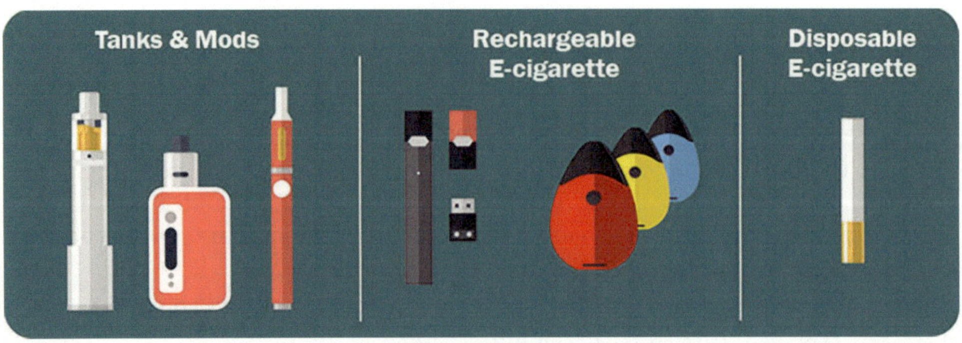

Figure 10.
E-cigarettes.

with nicotine, flavorings, and other chemicals. E-cigarettes produce vapor by heating the liquid. Smokers inhale this vapor of nicotine into their lungs. Nearby nonsmokers can also be exposed to this vapor when it is exhaled. Using an e-cigarette is sometimes called "vaping." It has been found that 4.4% of adults in Bangladesh are addicted to e-cigarettes with 5% males and 1.8% females [GATS, Bangladesh, 2017].

3. Passive smoking

Passive smoking causes due to secondhand tobacco exposure. It is also termed as Second-hand tobacco smoke (SHS), or environmental tobacco smoke. Passive smoking is the inhalation of tobacco smoke by nonsmoker. It occurs when the smoke drift from a lit cigarette or tobacco smoke exhaled by an active smoker in an environment and a nonsmoker nearby the active smoker inhales it. Many studies have revealed that exposure to SHS is linked to a number of noncommunicable health consequences among nonsmoker adults, including lung cancer, heart disease, and asthma [10], and among children including coughs and wheezing, acute lower respiratory infections, exacerbated asthma, middle ear infections, meningococcal meningitis, and sudden infant death syndrome [11–14]. GATS Bangladesh 2017 [5] has reported that 39.0% of adults were exposed to SHS at home, 42.7% of adults who worked indoors were exposed to SHS in enclosed areas at their workplace, 44.0% were exposed when using public transportation, 49.7% exposed while visiting restaurants, 12.7% exposed at health care facilities, 21.6% exposed at government buildings or offices, and 8.2% exposed to SHT at schools.

4. Tobacco use policies in workplaces and residences

Like many other countries, smoking is forbidden in enclosed public places and workplaces, with a slight exemption for restaurants with fewer walls in Bangladesh. But no clear smoking law is declared for residences. This produces a huge number of passive smokers, especially female and child passive smokers whose primary source of SHS exposure is in their own homes with at least one tobacco smoker. From GATS Bangladesh 2009, it has been found that among the female passive smokers, 21.4% were exposed in their residences and 18.9% were exposed at offices/workplaces [15]. The most common policy in home was that smoking was never allowed in home (30.97%), followed by no rules (29.82%), and smoking was allowed (22.15%). On the other hand, the most common policy in workplace was that smoking was prohibited (29.62%), followed by no rules (27.50%), and smoking was allowed (26.03%). However, 26.0% of passive tobacco smokers informed that smoking was allowed at their job place and 27.5% informed that there was no such smoking rule at the place.

5. Quitting methods

Besides various national strategies, some popular and useful quitting methods are also initiated to quit tobacco use, such as medications, nicotine replacement therapy, telephone helpline, counseling, etc. In two ways, prevalence of tobacco use can be minimized: (i) stopping initiation of new tobacco users, and (ii) quitting tobacco smoking. Successful quitting smoking is a continuous process, it may involve several attempts to quit and need to follow several methods. From GATS Bangladesh 2010, it has been found that among the tobacco smokers, 47.38% tried to quit smoking in the immediate past year of the survey [16]. Among them, 27.13% used anyone or compound form of quitting methods: 13.71% followed counseling, 0.76% followed nicotine replacement therapy, 0.57% followed traditional medication, 0.09% followed quitline or telephone helpline, 7.47% followed switching to smokeless tobacco, and 6.85% followed some other methods. Among the smokeless tobacco users, 31.89% tried to quit in the immediate past year of the survey. Among them, 24.83% used any one or compound form of quitting methods: 20.54% used counseling, 0.67% used nicotine replacement therapy, 0.54% used traditional medicine, 0.54% used quitline or telephone helpline, and 4.90% used other methods.

It has been found that male smokers, younger smokers, and smokers with lower wealth index were significantly and less likely to use one or more quitting methods at cessation attempts than their counterparts [16]. However, the study also investigated rural-urban inequities, educational inequities, and job inequities in using quitting methods. But, those were not found to be significant. The study also showed similar socio-demographic and economic behavior in using quitting methods to quit smokeless tobacco use.

6. Management of marketing and media coverage

Marketing and media play an important role in minimizing (or promoting) tobacco use. No doubt that the mass media and social media campaigns in the context of adverse effects of tobacco use can promote quitting or reducing tobacco smoking as well as smokeless tobacco use. On the other hand, advertisement of cigarette or *bidi* in mass media or in social media, signs promotion of *bidi* or cigarette, sponsorship of bidi or cigarette company in sports or sporting events, *bidi* or cigarette at sale price, free gifts, discount offers on other products, etc. may promote tobacco use and may initiate new users. Therefore, the Government and policymakers should monitor marketing and media coverage of tobacco products. A study found that 85.77% of adults noticed cigarette advertisements in the last 30 days of the survey [17]. The most common spot for observing cigarette advertisements was in a store (49.90%) and in other spots was 35.87%. In last 30 days of the survey, 2.07% noticed sport promotional events that encouraged tobacco users and 31.00% noticed other promotional events that encouraged them. It has also been found that 48.58% of people observed bidi advertisements. The most common spot for observing such advertisements was in stores (26.25%), and in other spots was 22.33%. Sport promotional events were observed by 0.65% of people and other promotional events were observed by 13.14% of people. The percentage of people who observed smokeless tobacco product advertisements was 22.49%. The most common spot was in a store (13.97%), and in other spots was (8.52%). Sport promotional event was observed by 0.21% and other promotional event was observed by 4.02% of people.

It has been identified that smokers, rural respondents, male respondents, younger respondents, higher educated respondents, and respondents with low-paid jobs or students were significantly and more likely to be inspired to smoke by observing such marketing policies for smoking-tobacco products. On the other hand, nonusers, rural respondents, male respondents, younger respondents, higher educated respondents, and respondents with middle economic status were significantly and more likely to be inspired to use by observing such marketing policy for smokeless-tobacco product.

7. Knowledge and attitude toward tobacco use

One of the most important strategies in reducing tobacco use prevalence is to increase knowledge about adverse effects of tobacco use in the population. It has been found that 94.8% of adults in Bangladesh know that tobacco smoking causes lung cancer, 89.5% know it causes heart attack, and 88.9% know it causes stroke [5]. On the other hand, 91.0% of adults know that smokeless tobacco use causes oral cancer, 82.5% know that it causes heart attack, and 82% know that it causes stroke. However, 93.1% of adults know that passive tobacco smoking causes serious illness. Another study has reported that female respondents are significantly less knowledgeable about the adverse effect of tobacco smoking and passive smoking [18]. Females are also less knowledgeable about the adverse effect of smokeless tobacco use but not statistically significant. Poorest people are significantly less knowledgeable about the adverse effect of passive smoking and smokeless tobacco use, and insignificantly less knowledgeable about tobacco smoking. Rural peoples are less knowledgeable about tobacco smoking, passive smoking, and smokeless tobacco use, but statistically insignificant. Respondents with less than secondary school completed are significantly more knowledgeable about the adverse effect of passive smoking and smokeless tobacco use than respondents with no formal schooling. Respondents with other educational levels are more knowledgeable but not statistically significant. However, education has not been found to play any significant role in the knowledge about the effect of tobacco smoking. Other common socio-demographic variables including age and profession are not significant to the knowledge about the effect of tobacco smoking, passive tobacco smoking, and smokeless tobacco use.

The study also analyzed tobacco use behavior of Bangladeshi respondents. It has been found that 11.48% of tobacco smokers smoke within 5 minutes after wakeup, 33.37% smoke between 6 and 30 minutes after wakeup, 25.37% smoke between 31 and 60 minutes after wakeup, and 29.54% smoke after one hour after wakeup [18]. Among the smokeless tobacco product users, 8.35% use within 5 minutes after wakeup, 25.30% use between 6 and 30 minutes after wakeup, 23.16% use between 31 and 60 minutes after wakeup, and 43.02% use after one hour after wakeup.

8. Discussion

Tobacco use, like many other addicted substances, is generally initiated as a result of an individual's social involvement with tobacco-using age-mates: The adolescent who is ready to access and living in a socio-cultural milieu attitudinally tolerant of tobacco use, in contrast to his or her nonuser, motivationally mature fellows, experiences the tremendous adjustive value of tobacco once overcoming its initial unpleasant consequences or side effects, Hence, initiation occurs almost without exception, from established users to novices, in a densely branched network.

In the cultural or endemic addictions, the intoxicant is socially accepted, e.g., smoking among males, and zarda with pan, sadapata, gul, etc. among females. Many studies reported that most of the addictions are initiated in late teens. However, 16 seemed to be the most common age according to the researchers.

The prevalence of tobacco smoking among adult males in Bangladesh is found to be very high and higher than neighboring countries like Pakistan [19] and Nepal [20], although lower than India [21]. It is hoped that tobacco smoking among females is not well accepted due to social customs in Bangladesh. But, large proportion of male smokers may cause passive smoking among females [22] as well as among children and nonsmoker males.

Smoking (or passive smoking) during gestation has long been linked to prenatal damage and subsequent antisocial behavior in adolescence. One study found that exposure to smoke was associated with increased psychopathology in offspring and that exposure to secondhand tobacco smoke during pregnancy predicted later conduct disorder [23]. Having a tobacco-smoking parent had a greater effect on behavior than other influences, including prematurity, low birth weight, and poor parenting practices. This in turn may be generated as an important component of ill-health causation. Therefore, the biosocial theory is highly tangled with tobacco use in sociology [24, 25]. As such, *public policy implications to trait theory* including family therapy, substance abuse hospitals, and mental health associations are helpful as *primary prevention programs*. However, services are dependent on the evidence that if a person's problems can be treated before they become devastating; some future smoking-related health problems can be prevented. *Secondary prevention programs* provide treatment such as psychological counseling to youths and adults who are at high risk of violating law of "smoking is prohibited in public places." *Tertiary prevention programs* may be a requirement of a visible amount of fine (say, tk 2000) to smoke first time at public places and gradually increase the amount of fine for the subsequent smoking at public places. More controversial has been the use of anti-smoking medications in fancy and fashionable packages. Some available antismoking medications in the world are Chantix, Bupropion, Topiramate, Naltrexone, Nicotine, Topamax, etc. Beximco Pharma Ltd. (BPL), Bangladesh's largest pharmaceutical company is manufacturing antismoking drug Zybex-SR (Bupropion Hydrochloride) since 2005.

Numerous psychologically based treatment methods range from individual counseling to behavior modification. Therapeutic interventions designed to make young adults better problem solvers may include methods that improve:

- coping and problem-solving abilities,
- relationships with peers, parents, and other juniors (or seniors),
- communication skills, and measures for resisting peer pressure,
- substantial thinking and decision-making skills,
- prosocial manners, including cooperation with others, self-responsibility, respecting elders, and public-speaking ability, and
- responsiveness.

E-cigarette is popular among teenagers (both males and females). E-cigarette is new in Bangladesh, but the prevalence is higher than in Japan [26]. British American Tobacco, Bangladesh first launched e-cigarettes in 2013 in Bangladesh [27]. Although the company overwhelming of its low-toxicants and fewer harmful substances compared to conventional cigarettes, the public health community has been divided over the possible benefits of e-cigarettes [28]. As it has been recently induced and its long-term effect has not been evaluated yet [29], the Government of Bangladesh should ban e-cigarettes. E-cigarette may not help in reduction of tobacco use; rather it will increase prevalence of the user.

Bangladesh is also a tobacco-cultivating country; the topmost is China, followed by India and Brazil [30]. Studies had identified that Company's incentives, profitability, guaranteed market for the tobacco crop, and economic viability encouraged farmers to cultivate tobacco [31] and sixty percent of household were found in shifting cultivation to tobacco in the last decade [32]. Government should also take some initiative to minimize tobacco cultivation.

9. Conclusion

Tobacco use not only affects health but also affects the user economically, which is enormous and upward. Due to its social acceptability and easy availability, more teenagers and young women are having access to it; some consider it as a part of their fashion and hence get addicted. As the effect of tobacco use is not immediate, very few people aim to quit. When the effect is visualized, it is too late to quit. Hence, successful cessation is lower. Some studies discussed the issues and challenges of tobacco control in Asia [33, 34] and policymakers should pay attention more keenly.

Therefore, besides strengthening the tobacco reduction acts, the government of Bangladesh should implement some infrastructure including establishment of smoking zones in educational institutions, government buildings/offices, and other crowded areas to reduce initiation of new users. Banning smoking in enclosed public places is not enough. Smoking should be banned in open crowded places, including "bus stoppage," train station, and public gatherings; in workplaces and home to minimize passive smoking. The government may prohibit attractive packaging and flavored tobacco products, and limit licensing retailers with number and location, especially nearby schools and colleges. In addition, government may take some initiative to renormalize the industries by continuously monitoring inclusion of child labor, and comprehensive banning advertisement, promotion, and sponsorship.

Conflict of interest

The author declares no conflict of interest.

Author details

Papia Sultana
Department of Statistics, University of Rajshahi, Rajshahi, Bangladesh

*Address all correspondence to: papia.stat@ru.ac.bd

References

[1] FAOSTAT 2018. Production Data. Available from: http://www.fao.org/faostat/en/#data. [Accessed: January 2, 2022]

[2] World Health Organization (WHO). Tobacco. 2020. https://www.who.int/en/news-room/fact-sheets/detail/tobacco. [Accessed: July7, 2020]

[3] Wu F, Chen Y, Parvez F, Segers S, Argos M, Islam T, et al. A prospective study of tobacco smoking and mortality in Bangladesh. PLoS One. 2013;**8**(3):e58516. DOI: 10.1371/journal.pone.0058516

[4] Tobacco control in Bangladesh: The tobacco epidemic. Available from: https://theunion.org/our-work/tobacco-control/bloomberg-initiative-to-reduce-tobacco-use-grants-program/tobacco-control-in-bangladesh. [Accessed: January 2, 2022]

[5] Fact Sheet: Global Adult Tobacco Survey (GATS) Bangladesh 2017. Available from: https://www.tobaccofreekids.org/assets/global/pdfs/en/Bangladesh_GATS_2017_factsheet.pdf. [Accessed: January 2, 2022]

[6] Rahman KMM, Tareque MI. Determinants of cigarette/bidi smoking among youth male in rural Mymensingh of Bangladesh: A cross-sectional study. PLoS One. 2020;**15**(12):e0244335. DOI: 10.1371/journal.pone.0244335

[7] Ahammed T, Ahmed NU, Uddin MJ. Changes in prevalence, and factors associated with tobacco use among Bangladeshi school students: Evidence from two nationally representative surveys. BMC Public Health. 2021;**21**:579

[8] Orellana-Barrios MA, Payne D, Mulkey Z, Nugent K. Electronic cigarettes-a narrative review for clinicians. The American Journal of Medicine. 2015;**128**(7):674-681. DOI: 10.1016/j.amjmed.2015.01.033

[9] Ki-Hyun K, Kabir E, Jahan SA. Review of electronic cigarettes as tobacco cigarette substitutes: Their potential human health impact. Journal of Environmental Science and Health, Part C. 2016;**34**(4):262-275. DOI: 10.1080/10590501.2016.1236604

[10] United States Department of Health and Human Services (USDHHS). The Health Consequences of Involuntary Exposure to Tobacco Smoke: A Report of the Surgeon General. Atlanta, GA: U.S: Department of Health and Human Services, Public Health Service, Centers for Disease Control; 2006

[11] Glantz SA, Parmley WW. Passive smoking and heart disease: Epidemiology, physiology, and biochemistry. Circulation. 1991;**83**:1-12. DOI: 10.1161/01.CIR.83.1.1

[12] National Cancer Institute. Health Effects of Exposure to Environmental Tobacco Smoke. Tobacco Control Monograph No. 10. Bethesda, MD: U.S. Department of Health and Human Services, National Institutes of Health, National Cancer Institute. NIH Pub No. 99-4645, 1999. Available at: http://cancercontrol.cancer.gov/brp/tcrb/monographs/monograph-10. [Accessed: December 12, 2013]

[13] Kriz P, Bobak M, Kriz B. Parental smoking, socioeconomic factors, and risk of invasive meningococcal disease in children: A population based case-control study. Archives of Disease in Childhood. 2000;**83**:117-121

[14] Hofhuis W, de Jongste JC, Merkus PJ. Adverse health effects of prenatal and postnatal tobacco smoke exposure

on children. Archives of Disease in Childhood. 2003;**88**:1086-1090

[15] Sultana P, Rahman MT, Roy DC, Akter S, Jung J, Rahman MM, et al. Tobacco control policies to promote awareness and smokefree environments in residence and workplace to reduce passive tobacco smoking in Bangladesh and its correlates. PLoS One. 2018;**13**(6):e0198942. DOI: 10.1371/journal.pone.0198942

[16] Sultana P, Alam J, Akter J, Kundu TR. Pattern of quitting methods used to promote tobacco cessation in Bangladesh and its correlates. Journal of Biometrics & Biostatistics. 2021;**12**:2

[17] Sultana P, Rahman MT, Roy DC. Marketing policy that accelerate tobacco use in Bangladesh: A statistical investigation. Journal of Biometrics & Biostatistics. 2017;**8**:386. DOI: 10.4172/2155-6180.1000386

[18] Rahman MT, Roy DC, Sultana P. Knowledge and attitude towards tobacco use in Bangladesh. Journal of Bangladesh Studies. 2016;**38**(2015):69-84

[19] Gilani SI, Leon DA. Prevalence and sociodemographic determinants of tobacco use among adults in Pakistan: Findings of a nationwide survey conducted in 2012. Population Health Matrics. 2013;**11**(16). DOI: 10.1186/1478-7954-11-16

[20] Sreeramareddy CT, Ramakrishnareddy N, Kumar HNH, Sathian B, Arokiasamy JT. Prevalence, distribution and correlates of tobacco smoking and chewing in Nepal: A secondary data analysis of Nepal Demographic and Health Survey-2006. *Substance Abuse Treatment, Prevention, and Policy*. 2012;**6**:33. DOI: 10.1186/1747X-6-33

[21] Mbulo L, Murty KS, Zhao L. Tobacco use and second hand smoke exposure among older adults in India. Journal of Aging and Health. 2021. DOI: 10.1177/08982643211000489

[22] Palupadi KM et al. Exposure to tobacco smoke among adults in Bangladesh. Indian Journal of Public Health. 2010;**55**(3):210-219

[23] Gatzke-Kopp LM, Theodore B. Direct and passive prenatal nicotine exposure and the development of externalizing psychopathology. Child Psychiatry and Human Development. 2007;**38**:255-269

[24] Adler-Mueller-Laufer-Grekul. Criminology. Canada: McGraw-Hill; 2008

[25] Siegel LJ. Criminology. Eleventh ed. USA: Senior Publisher; 2011

[26] Kuwabara Y, Kinjo A, Fujii M, Imamoto A, Osaki Y, Jike M, et al. Heat-not-burn tobacco, electronic cigarettes, and combustible cigarette use among Japanese adolescents: A nationwide population survey 2017. BMC Public Health. 2020;**20**:741. DOI: 10.1186/s12889-020-08916-x

[27] Vapour products. https://www.bat.com/ecigarettes#. [Accessed: April 4, 2022]

[28] Gilmore AB, Peeters S. Rapid response to Martin McKee's 'E-cigarettes and the marketing push that suprised everyone'. BMJ. 2013, 2013;**347**(f5780)

[29] Eaton DL, Kwan LY, Stratton KR. Public Health Consequences of E-Cigarettes. Washington, DC: National Academies Press; 2018

[30] Cook R. Ranking of countries that produce the most tobacco. 2022. https://

beef2live.com/story-ranking-countries-produce-tobacco-263-212893. [Accessed: April 11, 2022]

[31] Rahman MS, Ahmed NAMF, Ali M, Abedin MM, Islam MS. Determinant of tobacco cultivation in Bangladesh. Tobacco Control. 2020;**29**(6). DOI: 10.1136/tobacco control-2019-055167

[32] Motaleb MA, Irfanullah HM. Tobacco cultivation in Bangladesh: Is it a threat to traditional agro-practice? Indian Journal Traditional Knowledge. 2011;**10**(3): 481-485

[33] Mackay JM, Dorotheo EU, Assunta M, Ritthiphakdee B. Tobacco control in Asia-Pacific: Wins, challenges and targets. Tobacco Control. 2021;**2022**(31):146-149. DOI: 10.1136/tobaccocontrol-2021-056801

[34] Peeters S, Gilmore AB. Understanding the emergence of the tobacco industry's use of the term tobacco harm reduction in order to inform public health policy. Tobacco Control. 2014;**2015**(24):182-189. DOI: 10.1136/tobaccocontrol-2013-051502

Chapter 11

A Decision Support System for the Surgical Care during the Epidemic of Covid-19

Marwa Khalfalli and Jerome Verny

Abstract

Faced with the Covid epidemic, the optimization of human resources and materials is necessary to be able to treat as many victims as possible and to save them so as much as possible. Schedules are usually faced with a situation where new measures related to Covid are considered. This leads to higher risks and complications, especially in the preoperative service. Adapt the organization's surgical department for preserving their capacity and taking care of Covid and not Covid patients. To the best of our knowledge, the existing studies in the literature have treated the Covid scheduling task only on a service of the surgical process, mostly the preoperative service. In this study, we aim to design the keys of a new organization to preserve hospitalization capacities and ensure continuity of care, including all services of the surgery.

Keywords: covid surgical schedules, specialty, preoperative, operating rooms, postoperative, optimization, DSS

1. Introduction

The number of disasters has increased in recent decades in significant proportions. These disasters often result in a significant number of casualties requiring an urgent response. Faced with such a situation as the epidemic Covid, conventional and routine health means are often overtaken, and therefore is not effective to minimize this massive influx of victims.

The country has faced a new virus known as Corona Virus Disease 19 or Covid-19. Covid-19 spreads very quickly from person to person by contact. Covid-19 has resulted in our hospitals, and healthcare system is saturated by the number of critically ill people.

Hospitals are the mainstay of the care of severe Covid-19 patients; resuscitation service of the hugest hospitals have dozens of beds dedicated to the care of patients with Covid 19. Thus, the implementation of a system of hospital management conditioned by an optimization of the various medical resources is essential for patient safety. All actors in health facilities must be ready to face the health crisis generated by Covid-19.

Limiting the impact of Covid-19 care on scheduled and emergent activities must prevail during the rebound phase. The emergent cases must be limited as much as possible. The equity of access must be guaranteed to all patients. Thus, the burden related to Covid-19 must be shared equitably between the different territories and establishments. This principle should guide cooperation territorial and regional solidarity so as not to saturate a territory or an establishment and avoid inaccessibility to non-Covid care in these territories. The principle of territoriality of the adaptation of the hospital care must be driving the hospital response. Thus, within each territory, a declination operational regional principle must be carried out between hospital actors.

At the same time, they continue their indispensable activity for the care of the population. The particularity of the hospital system in exceptional situations is that it bases on the one hand on the emergency requiring decisions to be taken and quick actions to be carried out and, on the other hand, on the large number of victims to be treated in a short time. There is a lot of work that deals with organizational and optimization problems in hospital systems in normal circumstances. They are usually based on methods and tools from the manufacturing sector [1]. Most of this work is interested in the optimization of the operating room, which represents a bottleneck resource in the hospital system.

In the complex hospital, some departments have a lack of beds that will affect the quality of care, especially in the operating theater as the most sensitive department. Since the beginning of the crisis, there has been a lot of interest in the technical elements of patient care such as the positioning of patients in the supine position, artificial coma, but the functional and organizational changes are also very important.

To give all professionals, whether doctors or caregivers, the keys to a new organization to preserve hospitalization capacities and ensure continuity of care by:

- Strengthening as much as possible the upstream of the hospital sector as well as its alternatives to avoid any unnecessary hospitalization;

- Streamlining the path of hospitalized patients between conventional or scheduled stays, critical care (and no longer only in intensive care), and follow-up and rehabilitation care.

Units resuscitation made up of structures perennial, ephemeral, or upgraded, taking in charge of patients the most severe (intubation, failure extra-respiratory ...).

Intensive care service (Covid IC) consists of the structures of critical care outside resuscitation, welcoming Covid patients less severe (management noninvasive, mono defiance respiratory, ...).

Cooperation is encouraged between professionals (hospital and researchers) to ensure rehabilitation patients downstream of critical care, prevent and manage the post-resuscitation organization. Patients who have gone through the acute phase of the disease can be transferred to Covid IC, downstream of resuscitation. These health disasters of different natures and durations have resulted from the need to have a specific organization for service.

The care of Covid-19 patients has generated many changes in the organization of surgical services. In this chapter, we will study the impact of Covid on surgical care in the literature and design a complete decision support system for ensuring the continuity of surgical care during the epidemic of Covid-19.

2. Literature review

In this section, we will present the recent studies that proposed some solutions to manage the surgical cases in the Covid period. We will present the most recent studies in different surgery specialties: urologic, aortic, otorhinolaryngology and head and neck surgery, orthopedic, gynecologic, endocrine, maxillofacial, neurosurgical, and vascular service.

Tejido-Sánchez et al. [2] have modeled a care protocol to restart scheduled surgical activity in a Urology service of a third-level hospital in the Community of Madrid, in a safe way for the patients and professionals in the context of the Severe Acute Respiratory Syndrome Corona Virus 2 (SARS-CoV-2) epidemic. They have tested their protocol on 19 patients, 19 patients have been scheduled, of which two have been suspended for presenting Covid-19, one diagnosed by positive PCR for SARS-CoV-2, and another by laboratory and imaging findings compatible with this infection. No complications related to Covid-19 were detected after 10 days. That indicates that their proposed protocol ensures the correct application of preventive measures against the transmission of coronavirus infection is being safe and effective.

Covid-19.

To measure the impact of the delay of the programmed aortic surgeries during this epidemic, Perera et al. [3] have demonstrated that the death of 4.7% of postponed patients. Kail et al. [4] have discussed medical precautions required in the clinic, inpatient ward, and operation room of the otorhinolaryngology head and neck department, which aims to protect healthcare workers from Covid-19. While Sun et al. [5] have aimed to improve the success rate of treatment for otorhinolaryngology, head and neck surgery emergency surgeries and to reduce the SARS-CoV-2 infection rate in the perioperative period.

For the same objective of [3], M. Durand et al. [6] have dealt with the Covid conditions that allow the reporting of operations in the head and neck department. An analysis of reported patients is integrated into their studies.

In the orthopedic surgery department, Singh et al. [7] have determined the safety of elective, outpatient orthopedic sports procedures during the coronavirus pandemic at a high-volume orthopedic practice.

Piketty et al. [8] have focused on the new transformations generated by the Covid in the gynecologic department in the Foch hospital located in Paris, France. The authors have evaluated the surgery delays and their impacts on patients.

Kho et al. [9] have determined the incidence of perioperative coronavirus.

Disease in women undergoing benign gynecologic surgery and to evaluate perioperative complication rates in patients with active, previous, or no previous severe acute respiratory syndrome coronavirus 2 infections. Ozoner et al. [10] have proposed a comprehensive guide using existing guides and recommendations for reorganizing daily practice and the academic routine of neurosurgery during the Covid-19 pandemic. This study also aims to refine the substantial information for neurosurgical practice about this pandemic disease. Ermer et al. [11] have tracked endocrine surgery patients with treatment delays due to Covid-19 to investigate the relationship between Physician Assigned Priority Scoring (PAPS), the Medically Necessary, Time Sensitive (MeNTS) scoring system, and delay to surgery. Pagotto et al. [12] have evaluated the possible impacts of Covid-19 on oral and maxillofacial surgery practice, as well as the protocols employed by oral and maxillofacial surgeons to minimize the risks of contamination.

Also, Asghar [13] has considered indicators such as the presence of symptoms, characteristics of patients (age, sex, ...), and hospital data to study the results of the SARS test for oral-maxillofacial operations in 2020.

Among the addressed problems of the surgical department, the scheduling problem is a fundamental interest for the researchers because the scheduling task has a key role especially for the department having expensive resources. Thomson et al. [14] have cited several studies that approve the efficiency of hypo fractionated radiotherapy. They have evaluated the Covid changes on the surgery schedules to design a future complete database.

Güler et al. [15] have addressed the physician scheduling problem of a hospital during a Covid-19 pandemic. They have developed a Mixed-Integer Programming (MIP) model and embedded it into a spreadsheet-based Decision Support System (DSS).

In efforts to ensure adequate healthcare resource utilization, many electives or nonemergent surgical cases have been canceled since the coronavirus disease 2019 began, Dorash et al. [16] have analyzed the impact of the Covid-19 pandemic on surgical delays and adverse outcomes for patients with venous disease scheduled to undergo elective operations.

To the best of my knowledge, there is no quantitative study in the literature that considers the Covid policies in the whole surgical process. Authors are limited on one stage of the surgical process, as in [9], they have determined the incidence of perioperative coronavirus disease in women undergoing benign gynecologic surgery and to evaluate perioperative complication rates in patients with active, previous, or no previous severe acute respiratory syndrome coronavirus 2 infections.

Truche et al. [17] have quantified the surgical backlog during the Covid-19 pandemic in the Brazilian public health system and determined the relationship between state-level policy response and the degree of state-level delays in public surgical care.

Özkan et al. [18] have proposed a multicriteria optimization model while considering Intensive care unit admission for Covid-19-positive patients. The authors have used different methods to prioritize both criteria and patients, the Fuzzy Analytic Hierarchy Process (AHP) method to prioritize 19 criteria, and MULTIMOORA (**Multi**-Objective Optimization Based on a Ratio Analysis) is used to rank Covid-19-positive patients. They aim to find out which patient is more urgent for the intensive care unit.

Despite the added values of this research cited to optimize the scheduling tasks of surgical processes in the Covid period remains unresolved. it comes down to the continuous evolution of the epidemic and also to the complexity of the problem. In this study, we aim to design a global scheduling model of surgical processes in the Covid period while citing the different additional constraints compared with the traditional surgical process model.

3. COVID-19 operating room patient scheduling

3.1 Problem statement

We are considering the surgery scheduling problem whose objective is to assign an operating room and a one-day time slot to each programmed surgery. The operative process is triggered when a patient takes the appointment of surgical consultation and proceeds until exiting the hospital. This period is known in the scheduling theory as flow time. It breaks down into three-time services: the preoperative service, the per-operative service, and the postoperative service. The preoperative service corresponds to caring for patients until the day before surgery. The per-operative service is characterized by the duration of the surgery. The postoperative service covers all the care received by the patient after the surgery. In the preoperative service, the required resources are nurses, Pre-Holding (PH) beds while nurses and Post-Anesthesia Care (PAC)/Intensive Care Unit (IC) beds are involved in the postoperative service.

3.2 Perioperative management of surgical procedures during the Covid-19 pandemic

During Covid-19, new security and prevention measures are integrated into all stages of the surgical process, the operating rooms, and its facilities. Among these measures, a Covid test is required within three days of the operation date. This measure is applied to inpatients and outpatients, even if the patients do not have the Covid symptoms.

For patients who have a negative Covid test, their surgeries cannot be postponed and will be performed under prevention tools such as mask, spacing, respiratory protection, and reducing the access number to the OR and the staff exposure. For optimal use of human and material resources, operations can be grouped. Standard perioperative rules and transport procedures will have to be respected.

The consideration of the patient priority and urgency should be among the priorities of Covid surgical management.

3.2.1 Decision-making elements for performing surgery

Decisions to offer surgical treatment to the patient are made to ensure the absence of loss of chance in the treatment of each patient. Over-morbidity potential related to Covid-19 postoperative is part of the decision elements The order of programming is also taken in a multidisciplinary way, such as usually. This prioritization takes into account, among other things, the recommendations of up-to-date and available good practices, discussion with patients, impact on the patient's life expectancy or quality of life, the pathology involved, the context epidemic, and of course the possibilities of each surgeon (vacation). When the structure is not able to implement in the interest of the patient, surgical management within a time frame adapted to his situation must be considered to refer the patient to a structure able to ensure this care, thus allowing respect of the principle of access to care. To avoid any additional delays during these transfers of care, the structures are invited to organize themselves at the level territorial to prepare the management of this type of situation.

3.2.2 Proposals from surgical disciplines

Most disciplines have proposed a classification into four categories:

- Level 1: urgent care
- Level 2: coverage with the potential loss of chance if the postponement is greater than two or three months.

- Level 3: coverage with the potential loss of opportunity if the postponement of intervention is more than 6 months.

- Level 4: nonurgent care. Potential loss of opportunity if the postponement is more than 1 year

However, this classification may have justified postponing certain interventions by one month. Especially in oncology at the beginning of the white plan period. This means that these interventions can become priorities. The management of these patients can be carried out in another establishment if the blocks are not free at the level of the initial establishment.

In the current situation, the objective is to continue or even improve access to the management of surgical emergencies and "semi-emergencies," in proximity and at the level of the premises.

3.2.3 Conditions of support

A. Structures and premises:

In the current phase of the plateau of the epidemic and then that of degrowth, it will be necessary beforehand to determine at the regional and territorial level the volume of places resuscitation and beds or even Covid + blocks to keep. The reduction of the need for resuscitation beds will make it possible to regain conditions classic for surgical management in non-Covid units.

B. Situations:

- Outpatient care with the circuit in a UCA (Surgical Unit Ambulatory) to prioritize

- Conventional management with postoperative monitoring in PACU then in hospitalization (in room only in non-Covid units)

- Conventional management with postoperative monitoring in PACU then in intensive care and finally in hospitalization (in a room alone in the non-Covid units)

- Given the still partial knowledge about this epidemic, it is recommended to set up differentiated sectors (Covid and non-Covid) at the level of most institutions, while maintaining protective measures for caregivers and patients in all units.

C. Patients

They are informed by the surgeon and the anesthetist of the special conditions related to the Covid-19 pandemic, including the assessment of the risk/benefit balance of the intervention and the epidemic context at the time of the date of its intervention. The tracing in the patient's file of this information is essential.

They are also informed of symptoms suggestive of Covid-19 justifying contact with the surgical team and being able to postpone the surgical intervention.

Systematic contact the day before the intervention would be desirable with the same objective: determine a date of intervention and a place of care: specific Covid sector.

Screening for SARS-CoV-2 by RT-PCR of asymptomatic patients may be offered within 24/48 hours in preoperative, in case of:

- comorbidity at risk of a severe form of Covid-19,
- contact with a confirmed Covid-19 patient in the last 7 days,
- aerosol-generating surgeries,
- so-called major surgeries, at risk of severe form postoperatively (e.g., surgery),
- cardiac, abdominal, and heavy pelvic, organ transplantation, etc.).

Saliva samples may be more sensitive.

- In the case of positive sampling, the intervention will be postponed if possible, by 10 days.
- In the event of a confirmed intervention, with a positive sample, it is desirable to carry it out in a Covid+ sector.
- In case of emergency intervention, if the result of the sampling is not available, it is desirable to carry it out in a Covid+ sector.

Serological tests can be performed as soon as validated, and then certified tests are obtained by the competent authorities and integrated into care strategies. Computed Tomography (CT) scan of the chest can also be integrated into a strategy for analyzing the risk of contamination, particularly in case of emergency.

However, in adults, in the absence of availability of rapid biological testing, the performing a chest scan for lung damage silent in patients of unknown Covid status may be admissible in case emergencies (not allowing to wait for the results of the PCR) for another pathology, such as "Emergency surgical interventions, (ENT, oncology, etc.), ... "

D. Healthcare professionals

A serological test could be performed as soon as validated tests are obtained and then certified by the competent authorities and integrated into the arrangements for the assignment of staff, by the function of recommendations.

In the absence of immunization or the current period (pending validation of tests serological), a nasopharyngeal swab is performed for personnel symptomatic or contacts at risk, a nasopharyngeal swab is performed for personnel symptomatic or contacts at risk. If the sample is positive, an isolation measure is taken following national recommendations.

Pending the availability of all validated and certified biological tests, the instructions regarding the personal protective equipment of caregivers remain unchanged.

3.3 Constraints

The OR scheduling problem treated in this study includes all the services of the surgical process. Our model includes the most constraints in the real-life operating room department. Additional constraints related to the Covid policies will be presented also.

We assume various realistic procedures:

- In the surgical process, the patient flow includes three services without waiting time between them
- A unit service cannot be interrupted before its end
- Same priority for all patients
- The operating rooms are uniforms
- There is no ordering constraint between services of different operations
- The duration of each service is a deterministic parameter
- The transfer time between the services of an operation is determined under Covid policies
- The setup time is considerable under Covid policies

The following constraints are considered in the optimization model:

No-wait in the surgical process: The operating theater includes beds in PH service, operating rooms, and beds in PAC or IC services. Each patient must first pass through a bed of PH service and then into an operating room and then through a bed of PAC/IC services without waiting time between these three units.

Resources type: The resources of operating theater are classified into several types according to the resources required by the operation.

Operation type: Three types of operation: small, large, and extra-large, this classification depends on the length of the operation duration. The operating times for each service were defined as follows: the duration of the preoperative service is fixed for all operations, and similarly the duration of the postoperative service is fixed for all operations. The duration of the preoperative service is different on the operation type.

Requirement compatibility of operation and operation specialty: we have considered several operation specialties in the model and consequently different surgeon specialties are presented.

Availability of surgeons: Ensure the availability of the assigned surgeon.

Resource number: The number of resources required on resource type C must exactly be equal to the assigned resources to perform the surgery i in the service j.

In our model, we consider the followings sets, parameters, and decisions variables.

I: All operations, $i = 1..N$.

JO_i: All services of operation$i$, $JO_i = \{1, 2, 3\}$, $i = 1..N$.

P: All operation specialties, $p \in P$.

C: 0peration complexity$c$, C= {1: difficult; 2: easy}, $c \in C$.

S: Elements of resources. $s=$ {professor surgeon, resident surgeon, assistant surgeon, anesthesiologist, nurse, anesthetist, OR, PH bed, and PAC bed}.

JR_s: operation services that can be treated by resources, $s \in S$.

n^s_{ij}: The required resource s for treating operation i at service j. $i \in I, j = 1, 2, 3, s \in S$.

T^s_{ij}: The duration of operation i at service j by resources. $i \in I, j = 1, 2, 3, s \in S$.

TW^t_S: The availability of resource s. $TW^t_S = \left[STW^t_S, ETW^t_s\right]$ where STW^t_S and ETW^t_s are consecutively the start time and the end time of the time window t, $t \in N$, $t \leq |TW_s|$.

M: A large positive number.

RT_1: Working time of doctors.

RT_2: Working time of anesthetists and nurses.

R^s_{ij}: The availability of resource s during service j of operation i. $R^s_{ij} = 1$ if the resource s is available, $R^s_{ij} = 0$ otherwise. $i \in I, j = 1, 2, 3, s \in S$.

B^i_{pc}: =1 if an operation i is suitable to specialty p and complexity c, B^i_{pc}=0 otherwise, $i \in I; p \in P$.

Q^s_{pc}: =1 if a resources can treat the operation in its specialty p and complexity c, Q^s_{pc}=0 otherwise. $s \in S$.

ST_{ij}: Beginning of operation i, $i \in I, j = 1, 2, 3$.

CT_{ij}: End of operation i at service j, $i \in I, j = 1, 2, 3, s \in S$.

X^s_{ij}: =1 if resource s is assigned to operation i at service j, X^s_{ij}=0 otherwise, $i \in I, j = 1, 2, 3; s \in S$.

$A_{aa'}$: =1 if operation stage a occurs before operation stage a' requiring the same resource, $A_{aa'} = 0$ otherwise, $a, a' \in J_s$.

$y^i_{aa'}$: For the same operation i, $y^i_{aa'}$=1 if its service a precedes service a', $y^i_{aa'}$=0 otherwise. a, a' $\in J_i$, $i \in I$.

v^{st}_{ij}: =1 if resource s performs operation i at service j within its available time window TW^t_s, v^{st}_{ij} =0 otherwise. $i \in I, j = 1, 2, 3; s \in S; t \in [1, |TW_s|]$

$$CT_{ij} = ST_{ij} + \max_{s \in S}\left\{T^s_{ij}.X^s_{ij}\right\}; \quad i \in I, \; j = 1, 2, 3 \tag{1}$$

$$CT_{ij} = ST_{i(\;j+1)}, \quad i \in I; j = 1, 2 \tag{2}$$

$$CT_{ia'} - CT_{ia} \geq \max_{s \in S} T^s_{ia'} - M\left(1 - y^i_{aa'}\right), \quad a < a'; i \in I; \quad a, a' \in JO_i \tag{3}$$

$$CT_{ia} - CT_{ia'} \geq \max_{s \in S} T^s_{ia} - My^i_{aa'}), \quad i \in I; a, a' \in JO_i; a < a' \tag{4}$$

$$CT_{i'a'} - CT_{ia} \geq \max_{s \in S} T^s_{i'a'} - M(1 - A_{aa'}); \quad i, i' \in I, \quad i \neq i'; a, a' \in JR_s \tag{5}$$

$$CT_{ia} - CT_{i'a'} \geq \max_{s \in S} T^s_{ia} - MA_{aa'}; i, i' \in I, \quad i \neq i'; \quad a, a' \in JR_s \tag{6}$$

$$\sum_{s \in S} X^s_{ij}.R^s_{ij} = n^s_{ij}; \quad i \in I, \; j = 1, 2, 3 \tag{7}$$

$$\sum_{c \in C}\sum_{p \in P} B^i_{pc}.Q^s_{pc} \geq X^s_{ij}; \quad i \in I, \; j = 1, 2, 3; \quad s \in S \cap \{1, 2, \; 3\} \tag{8}$$

$$X^s_{ij}.\sum_{t=1}^{|TW_s|}\left(v^{st}_{ij}.STW^t_s\right) \leq ST_{ij}; \quad i \in I, \; j = 1, 2, 3; s \in S \tag{9}$$

$$X_{ij}^{s}.\sum_{t=1}^{|TWs|}\left(v_{ij}^{st}.ETW_{s}^{t}\right)\geq CT_{ij}^{s};\quad i\in I,\ j=1,2,3;\ s\in S \tag{10}$$

$$ST_{i1}\geq 0,\quad i\in I \tag{11}$$

$$\sum_{s\in S}X_{ij}^{s}=1;\qquad i\in I,\ j=1,2,3 \tag{12}$$

$$X_{ij}^{s}\in\{0,1\}\qquad i\in I,j=1,2,3;\ s\in S \tag{13}$$

$$y_{aa'}^{i}\in\{0,1\}\qquad i\in I;a,a'\in JO_{i} \tag{14}$$

$$A_{aa'}\in\{0,1\}\quad a,a'\in JR_{s} \tag{15}$$

Equation (1) calculates the end time of operation *iat* service *j*. Equation (2) defines that the end of operation *i* at service *j* is the beginning of stage *j + 1* of operation *i* (no-wait). Equations (3) and (4) indicate that two services of an operation *i* should not be treated at the same time. Equations (5) and (6) determine that a resource s can be only assigned to one operation service simultaneously. Equation (7) means that the assigned resource should conform to the necessary resources to operat*e i at* service *j*. Equation (8) means that the assigned surgeon has the required proficiency required by the operation specialty and complexity. Equations (9) and (10) mean that the operation must be performed during the available time windows of its assigned resources. Equation (11) means that all operations beginning equal to or superior to time 0. Equation (12) indicates that an operation must be treated once only. Equations (13) to (1) are binary variables.

To obtain a Covid optimization model that includes all the services of the surgical process and all specialties, the following constraints are added in the optimization model:

- No surgeries were performed without PCR results
- Only patients with negative test results were operated on
- Patients with positive signs were canceled and asked to come for a PCR test. Singh et al. [7] have approved that 3.5% of patients tested positive for Covid-19 and were significantly younger when compared with patients testing negative. As of April 3, all scheduled patients received a PCR test in the hospital on the eve of surgery.
- Patients whose operation was postponed were contacted by the department secretaries and physicians during the 4 months following the study period. After five unsuccessful calls, patients were deemed lost to follow-up.
- Management of asymptomatic or confirmed Covid-19+ patient. If possible, it is best to postpone the intervention 7–10 days after the end of symptoms.
- Preference should be given to an outpatient intervention.
- The need for a large quantity of special equipment to ensure personal protection such as masks, gels, ... these products are very necessary for the healthcare

providers especially in the most affected areas by Covid-19. Unfortunately, they are not always available with the necessary quantities.

- Healthcare staff must do the necessary precautions to protect against the transmission of Covid-19 from patients.
- Patients who are attracted by Covid-19 were usually hospitalized and needed the care of healthcare workers.
- The Covid patients are more prior than the elective patients to use the ORs that integrate breathing machines.
- For safety, and to ensure that resources, hospital beds, and equipment are available to patients critically ill with Covid-19, non-emergency procedures be delayed. Factors will influence whether the operation should be done now or delayed. They will include the extent of Covid-19 including the hospital's capacity.

4. Conclusions

As pandemic Covid-19 dynamically changes in our society, it is important to consider how the pandemic has affected the schedules of surgical operations. To develop a complete surgical scheduling model integrating Covid policies, we aim to identify additional constraints in all stages of the surgical process that could be used to inform practice and policy for future pandemics and disasters. This study could be the pioneer for global optimization of surgical service during the epidemic. This search provides for the initiation of several specific procedures on the part of the nursing and administrative staff with a minimum of modification of the traditional hospital organization. But these forecasts must be adapted to cultural conditions and specific economic means. This search can be considered the pioneer of future optimization models that consider the complete Covid surgical process. Organizations continue to prepare recommendations for physicians treating patients including those with cancer. The physicians treating you are meeting in teams to guide ongoing care. Care options may include other treatments while waiting for a safe time to proceed with surgery.

Author details

Marwa Khalfalli[1*] and Jerome Verny[2]

1 HF-LAB, Paris, France

2 Noema Business School, Rouen, France

*Address all correspondence to: marwa.khalfalli@highfi.net

References

[1] Chaabane S, Guinet A, Smolski N, Guiraud M, Luquet B, Actas Urológicas Españolas Marcon E, et al. Industrial management and management of operating theatres. Annales French Annales of Anesthesia and Resuscitation Françaises. 2002;**22**:904–908

[2] Tejido-Sánchez A, González-Díaz A, García-Rojo R, Santos-Pérez de la Blanca R, Varela-Rodríguez C, Ruiz-López PA, et al. Design of an assistance protocol for the restart of scheduled urologic surgery in a COVID-19 epidemic period. Diseño de un protocolo asistencial para el reinicio de la cirugía urológica programada en periodo de epidemia COVID-19. 2020;**44**:597-603. DOI: 10.1016/j.acuroe.2020.10.005

[3] Perera K, Wohlauer MV, D'Oria M, Savlania A, Bath J, Colborn K, et al. Impact of COVID-19 on patients scheduled for aortic surgery. Journal of Vascular Surgery. 2021;**74**:e52. DOI: 10.1016/j.jvs.2021.06.086

[4] Kai X, Xiaoquan L, Zheng L. Suggestions on the prevention of COVID-19 for health care workers in department of otorhinolaryngology head and neck surgery. World Journal of Otorhinolaryngology - Head and Neck Surgery. 2020;**6**:S2-S5. DOI: 10.1016/j.wjorl.2020.03.002

[5] Sun Y, Zhang L, Cheng Q, Hu Y, Xiao H. Diagnosis and treatment of emergency surgeries in otorhinolaryngology, head and neck surgery during the covid-19 outbreak: A single center experience. World Journal of Otorhinolaryngology - Head and Neck Surgery. 2020;**6**:S16-S21. DOI: 10.1016/j.wjorl.2020.05.002

[6] Durand M, Mirghani H, Bonfils P, Laccourreye O. Surgery under COVID: An observational study. European Annals of Otorhinolaryngology, Head and Neck Diseases. 2021; DOI: 10.1016/j.anorl.2021.06.003

[7] Singh H, Isak I, Knapik DM, Vadhera AS, Gursoy S, Cole BJ, et al. No patients having elective outpatient orthopaedic surgery performed in an ambulatory surgery center using preoperative screening protocols during the coronavirus pandemic developed COVID-19. Arthroscopy, Sports Medicine, and Rehabilitation. 2021;**3**(4): e1141–e1146. DOI: 10.1016/j.asmr.2021.05.001

[8] Piketty J, Carbonnel M, Murtada R, Revaux A, Asmar J, Favre-Inhofer A, et al. Collateral damage of COVID-19 pandemic: The impact on a gynecologic surgery department. Journal of Gynecology Obstetrics and Human Reproduction. 2022;**51**(1):102255. DOI: 10.1016/j.jogoh.2021.102255

[9] Kho RM, Chang OH, Hare A, Schaffer J, Hamner J, Northington GM, et al. Surgical outcomes in benign gynecologic surgery patients during the COVID-19 pandemic (SOCOVID study). Journal of Minimally Invasive Gynecology. 2022;**29**(2):274-283. DOI: 10.1016/j.jmig.2021.08.011

[10] Ozoner B, Gungor A, Hasanov T, OrkunToktas Z, Kilic T. Neurosurgical practice during coronavirus disease 2019 (COVID-19) pandemic. World Neurosurgery. 2020;**140**:198-207. DOI: 10.1016/j.wneu.2020.05.195

[11] Ermer JP, JMS B, Go BC, Philipson B, Gabriel PE, Pryma DA, et al. Endocrine surgical procedures during COVID-19: Patient prioritization and time to surgery. Journal of Surgical Research.

2021;**268**:459-464. DOI: 10.1016/j.jss.2021.07.006

[12] Pagotto L, Santos T, Pastore G. Impact of COVID-19 on maxillofacial surgery practice: A systematic review. Brazilian Journal of Otorhinolaryngology. 2021. DOI: 10.1016/j.bjorl.2021.09.002

[13] Asghar M. Hematological characteristics of patients in coronavrius 19 infection: A systematic review and meta-analysis. Journal of Community Hospital Internal Medicine Perspectives. 2020;**10**:508-513

[14] Thomson DJ, Yom SS, Saeed H, El Naqa I, Ballas L, Bentzen SM. et al. Radiation fractionation schedules published during the COVID-19 pandemic: A systematic review of the quality of evidence and recommendations for future development. International Journal of Radiation Oncology Biology Physics. 2020;**108**(2):379–389. DOI: 10.1016/j.ijrobp.2020.06.054

[15] Güler M, Geçici E. A decision support system for scheduling the shifts of physicians during COVID-19 pandemic. Computers & Industrial Eng ineering. 2020;**150**:106874. DOI:10.1016/j.cie.2020.106874

[16] Dorosh J, Wohlauer M, Kabeil MD, Malgor R, AnnO'Banion L, Lopez-Pena G, et al. Impact of COVID-19 on patients undergoing scheduled operations for venous disease. Journal of Vascular Surgery. 2021;**74**:e266.DOI: 10.1016/j.jvs.2021.06.390

[17] Truche P, NunesCampos L, BarrozoMarrazzo E, GerkRangel A, Bernardino R, Nbowder A, et al. Association between government policy and delays in emergent and elective surgical care during the COVID-19 pandemic in Brazil: A modeling study. The Lancet Regional Health – America. 2021;**3**:100056. DOI: 10.1016/j.lana.2021.100056

[18] Özkan B, Özceylan E, Kabak M, UğraşDikmen A. Evaluation of criteriaéà and COVID-19 patients for intensive care unit admission in the era of pandemic: A multi-criteria decision making approach. Computer Methods and Programs in Biomedicine. 2021;**209**:106348. DOI: 10.1016/j.cmpb.2021.106348

Chapter 12

The Well-Being of Doctors during the COVID-19 Pandemic

Dabota Yvonne Buowari

Abstract

The COVID-19 pandemic has ravaged the world, and the world is trying to adapt to the new world. Healthcare workers had to undergo stress in order to combat the pandemic. Doctors worked hard even with the several restrictions on movement, such as curfews and lockdowns. Doctors still had to go to work. The work of doctors is stressful, and this is made worse by the COVID-19 pandemic. The pandemic has led to a poor well-being of doctors. Doctors are now exposed to several mental health disorders such as depression, burnout, insomnia and poor physical, psychological, psychosocial, and mental well-being. Well-being of doctors during the COVID-19 pandemic is a study that deals with the well-being of health workers in general, and doctors in particular, and is important and original in the field. Hospital managers and employers should develop strategies to reduce burnout in doctors and improve their well-being. This includes provision of counseling services and vacation for doctors.

Keywords: well-being, COVID-19, physicians, mental health, psychological well-being

1. Introduction

The COVID-19 pandemic, which emerged in China in December 2019, has spread to several countries on every continent globally. Initially, several measures were taken to control the novel virus with continuous research and the invention of a vaccine. There has been a rise in the number of disasters that have occurred including epidemics and pandemics worldwide. When these occur, the worst affected professionals are healthcare workers as they are in the frontline fighting against emerging and reemerging diseases and microorganisms [1].

Healthcare workers including doctors are involved in combating the COVID-19 pandemic as the role they have been involved in cannot be overemphasized, and this has caused more burden for them in addition to their previous regular work [2–5]. Other categories of healthcare workers are also at the forefront in the fight to bring the COVID-19 pandemic to an end such as nurses, laboratory technologists, technicians and scientists, medical urologists, pathologists, medical microbiologists, pharmacists, hospital/health assistants, and orderlies, paramedic including other hospital support staff such as ambulance drivers, medical record officers. In recent times, one of the pandemics that has hit the human race with detrimental effects on healthcare and also led to a crisis in the economy of several countries is the COVID-19 pandemic [6, 7].

Since healthcare workers are at the forefront in the fight against the COVID-19 pandemic and they are also involved in the treatment of patients infected with the severe acute respiratory distress coronavirus-2, they are at the risk of being infected with the novel virus; therefore, they are at risk of losing their lives to this novel virus [3, 6, 8]. The outburst of the COVID-19 pandemic globally has impacted negatively on healthcare systems due to the challenges it has created in health care [9]. Before the COVID-19 pandemic, medical care is provided for individuals that are ill by healthcare professionals including physicians and nurses [10]. This care provided by doctors and nurses has continued during the COVID-19 pandemic. It can be stressful and sometimes terrifying as healthcare workers continue providing medical care for patients during a pandemic [4]. The occupation of medical practitioners is stressful and different doctors have diverse ways of coping [11]. Healthcare workers are exposed to several challenges during the COVID-19 pandemic [12].

Healthcare professionals may contract infections at the workplace (nosocomial infections) even during epidemics and pandemics, and they can also serve as carriers of such infections. Subsequently, psychological distress may occur [13]. Globally, the COVID-19 pandemic has impacted negatively on the well-being and mental health affecting emotions, and it is of great concern [14]. The stressful nature of providing medical care for patients infected with the severe acute respiratory coronavirus-2 lightens the already increased level of burnout and other psychological symptoms experienced by healthcare professional [15]. During this COVID-19 pandemic, healthcare professionals are risking their lives they are on the frontline in the fight against the pandemic as they are the first responders [6]. Several strategies are been taken to provide support for healthcare professionals during the COVID-19 pandemic at different levels both individually and also at the organizational level [15].

1.1 The COVID-19 pandemic

The COVID-19 pandemic started in the Wuhan town in the Hubei Province of China in December 2019. All the first set of patients who had the illness had visited an animal market; hence, it was relieved that the carrier of the causative virus was the fruit bat. There were speculations that the causative virus, which was identified to be a coronavirus, emerged from the animal market; hence, the market was later closed down. Before this time there have been outbreaks of disease caused by coronaviruses leading to the epidermis. In the twenty-first century, the pandemic caused by COVID-19 is the worst that has been experienced by mankind [6, 16].

A coronavirus is a group of viruses that belong to the family *Coronaviridae.* They infect both animals and humans [3]. The causative coronavirus of the COVID-19 pandemic when it was reported first in Wuhan, China, was named 2019 novel coronavirus (2009-nCoV) in December 2019 [17]. The virus was later renamed severe acute respiratory syndrome coronavirus-2 (SARS-CoV-2) and the disease coronavirus disease 2019 (COVID-19) [18]. Within a very short time due to the interaction between human beings, migration, and travels, the virus spread to several countries on every continent worldwide [2, 8, 17, 18].

It was declared a pandemic and a public health emergency of international concern by the World Health Organization in January 2020 [18–20]. Pandemics consume the time of healthcare professionals as they care for their patients, hence leading to a global crisis [21]. Before the emergence of SARS-CoV-2, three other deadly outbreaks have been experienced by mankind in the twenty-first century caused by novel coronavirus [22]; the novel viruses are the Severe Acute Respiratory Syndrome

Coronavirus (SARS-CoV) and the Middle East Respiratory Syndrome Coronavirus (MERS-CoV) [3, 18, 22]. These novel coronaviruses attack the respiratory system leading to acute respiratory infections and are contracted by close human-to-human contact since they are contagious, hence leading to the death of a large number of people in a very short time [3, 8, 22].

1.2 What is well-being and its importance

There is no definitive definition for well-being [21, 23]. There are different forms of well-being, which include physical, psychological, and mental well-being. Therefore, every employer must provide a safe workplace for the employees to be of good well-being. Also, individuals to some extent are responsible for their well-being as negative well-being will affect the health of the person; strategies that support the psychological well-being are beneficial to physicians, and it is necessary for them to feel safe at all times, especially during an epidemic or pandemic [24]. Poor well-being can lead to burnout and distress. Good well-being is also necessary as it helps healthcare workers against nosocomial infections to improve the psychological well-being of doctors, they must be supported continuously, especially by their managers. The well-being of doctors has been investigated in several publications. The term "well-being" is often used to illustrate the state of a person or group of people concerning their financial resources psychosocial, psychological, health, and spirituality [25]. The well-being of doctors is important, that is why it is stated in the physicians' pledge, which every doctor recites at the time of induction into medical practice. The physician's pledge states that "I will attend to my health, mental well-being and abilities to provide care of the highest standard" [26]. This means that the mental health and well-being of the physicians are very important; the physicians need to have stable mental well-being to function effectively. The word "well-being" is also included in the definition of health by the World Health Organization, which defines health as a state of complete physical mental and social well-being and not merely the absence of disease or infirmity [27]. The components of well-being are physical, mental, emotional, cultural, psychological, and psychosocial health. The occupation of physicians is stressful, and they sometimes work under pressure beyond their control [28]. There is a positive relationship between well-being and quality of life in addition to job satisfaction [10, 25], especially psychological well-being; therefore, all aspects of the well-being of doctors need special attention [1, 28]. To understand it better and identify critical areas of utmost need. Burnout is an outcome of poor well-being.

1.3 Impact of the COVID-19 pandemic on doctors

The COVID-19 pandemic has impacted negatively on every aspect of life and professions including healthcare [16]. It has several impacts on healthcare professionals and their well-being. This is worsened by the risk of contracting the novel virus in the medical workplace because of the health problems caused by the SARS-CoV-2, which has led to increased stress levels in healthcare workers including doctors [2, 6, 8, 15, 29–33]. The mental health of physicians who have been affected by the COVID-19 pandemic needs to be identified by employers [29]. The mental health of physicians has been affected by the COVID-19 pandemic [16].

The impact of the pandemic is worst on healthcare professionals including doctors because they are on the frontline and as such are exposed directly to the virus in the course of their work [3, 6]. Besides stress, other impacts of the COVID-19 pandemic on doctors are [3, 6, 7, 13, 16, 21, 30, 33–35]:

1. Anxiety
2. Exposure to the severe acute respiratory distress syndrome coronavirus-2 (SARS-CoV-2)
3. Long working hours
4. Psychological problems especially distress
5. Tiredness and fatigue
6. Burnout
7. Stigmatization
8. Violence at the workplace can be physical or psychological
9. Depression
10. Disturbance in sleep pattern
11. Panic
12. Isolation and seclusion
13. Exhaustion especially emotionally [34]
14. Poor job satisfaction [34]

The pandemic has also affected healthcare financial and resources [2]. All professions related to healthcare are stressful, and this has been made worst by the COVID-19 pandemic [15]. According to the British Medical Association (BMA), 45% of physicians previously diagnosed with depression, stress, anxiety, and burnout, and other mental health disorders before the COVID-19 pandemic have developed worsened symptoms [36].

Worldwide, there has been a notable burden of the COVID-19 pandemic [32]. Fear of contracting the COVID-19 pandemic is highest in the health sector [35]. Therefore, healthcare professionals need to be supported to ameliorate the impact of the COVID-19 pandemic [37]. As some of these impacts of the COVID-19 pandemic can affect the well-being of doctors leading to medical errors, litigation, consideration of exiting the medical profession and even mental and physical ill-health.

1.4 The well-being of doctors before the COVID-19 pandemic

Meeting full potential and having the feeling of a positive nature make up for well-being. Their well-being is very important for their mental health and physical health [23]. Well-being affects the quality of life; therefore, well-being of doctors' affects job satisfaction, the prognosis of a patient's illness, and the physicians' health [38]. This is because the well-being of a doctor will affect the way they relate to their patient and also carry out their work. The improvement of well-being is necessary for every workplace [39]. Poor well-being of doctors can lead to burnout, which in turn leads to medical errors, poor job satisfaction, poor quality of the care rendered, and increased cost of well-being [39]. This exposes the physician to litigation as the clients/patients will not understand the stressful nature of the doctor's work.

Doctors are trained not to care for themselves, even their well-being but to care for their patients in times of emergencies [35]. Doctors' well-being has been investigated globally even in times of crisis and health emergencies [32], and it has been found that doctors have poor well-being. The risk factors that can lead to poor well-being of doctors can be divided into two, which can be due to the individual or occupational factors. The individual risk factors include personality traits and psychological and psychosocial factors; psychological distress can occur when the individual factors interact with occupational factors. The occupational risk factors are doctors directed related to the work, which can be the various aspects of the healthcare job, which may be clinical or structural [28].

1.5 Impact of the COVID-19 pandemic on the well-being of doctors

The COVID-19 pandemic has created a lot of negative impacts on medical doctors and also on other categories of healthcare professionals. It has led to poor well-being of physicians evidenced by several studies conducted on the impact of the COVID-19 pandemic on the mental health and well-being of doctors before the pandemic, doctors have suffered burnout and stress due to the nature of their work [33]. This is now worse than the COVID-19 pandemic. Doctors and medical students must be supported as this will improve their psychological, psychosocial, mental, and physical a minority as long as the COVID-19 pandemic lasts [36, 37]. There have been an exacerbation and dilemma between the ethics guiding the medical profession and the pressure caused by the COVID-19 pandemic [37]. Doctors need to know their breaking point and limitations so that they do not develop symptoms of burnout at their workplace [7, 37].

Besides poor well-being, other impacts of the COVID-19 pandemic on doctors are anxiety, burnout, depression, distress, exhaustion, and sleep deprivation [21]. During the outbreak of infectious disease, either as an epidemic or pandemic, the way doctors respond to it psychologically is complicated, and it also varies [40]. The healthcare profession is the worst hit among all professions by the COVID-19 pandemic because healthcare professionals come directly in contact with individuals infected with SARS-CoV-2 [16, 31, 41]. The COVID-19 pandemic is a cause of anxiety, stress, burnout, and depression among physicians [4, 16, 41, 42]. This is because the work of physicians involves caring for sick persons. Even during health emergencies, epidemics, and pandemics, physicians continue in their job as there is no half despite the pandemic caused by an infectious disease [4]. Globally, the physical and mental well-being of physicians is challenged by the coronavirus disease-2019 (COVID-19) pandemic [43].

Due to the negative impact of the COVID-19 pandemic on the well-being of doctors and other healthcare professionals, the World Health Organization (WHO) compiles healthcare workers to safeguard their well-being especially their mental health and psychological well-being [19]. Therefore, it is necessary that physicians and their employers take steps to improve the well-being of physicians. Physicians must take several precautionary measures at their workplace in order not to contract the SARS-CoV-2, it is also that they also manage their mental health and psychological well-being [19].

Helpful coping strategies should be adapted, and unhelpful ones should be discarded such as recreational drugs, alcohol, and tobacco [19]. This is because these harmful substances will cause addiction and affect physical health. They will also worsen mental health. It is necessary to identify and protect the various causes of poor well-being of doctors during the COVID-19 pandemic to combat and mitigate them [8, 43].

However, there is a lack of interventions that protect the well-being, especially the mental health of physicians during the COVID-19 pandemic that is evidence-based [19]. Some coping strategies that can be adopted to protect and preserve the well-being of doctors during the COVID-19 pandemic are self-assistance, self-belief ability to cope, and support from the employer and organization [41]. Physicians will teach their full potential and carry out their work dutifully during the COVID-19 pandemic when their mental health is preserved, and they are prevented from anxiety, stress, and depression during the health emergency [19].

1.6 Factors and sources of poor well-being of doctors during the COVID-19 pandemic

Poor well-being at the workplace leads to several consequences, and this has been made worst by the COVID-19 pandemic [43]:

1. Stigmatization

2. Discrimination from family members because the doctors may be a source of infection [31, 38].

3. Working on the frontline: This is a challenge because they are in direct contact with patients who are already infected with the deadly virus [5, 38, 40–44]. It is evidenced by a study by Veeraragharan and Srimivasan [42].

4. Change in work schedule: The COVID-19 pandemic has led to the disarray of the work schedule of doctors. They are now working long hours, and they are also burdened with increased workload [5, 7, 13, 38, 40, 42]. These increased working hours have led to sleep deprivation and work-life imbalance [16] and a heavy workload [5].

5. Shortage of medical supplies: The COVID-19 pandemic has led to a shortage of medical supplies globally [38, 42].

6. Lack of training on the use and availability of personal protective equipment: Personal protective equipment is very important during the COVID-19 pandemic to protect doctors and other healthcare professionals. It is supposed to be worn during the pandemic, but this is not the case in all medical settings sometimes when it is available, the doctors are not trained on how it should be used properly. This is a source of poor well-being during the COVID-19 pandemic [8, 16, 38, 44]. The personal protective equipment causes dehydration and tiredness when it is worn [2].

7. Female gender: From various studies, the mental health of female healthcare workers is the worst affected [7, 8, 39].

8. Lack of incentives: Some governments gave financial incentives to their healthcare workers during the COVID-19 pandemic because of the risk and exposure while caring for the sick during the COVID-19 pandemic [8, 38].

9. Fear of contracting SARS-CoV-2: There is great fear of contracting the novel SARS-CoV-2 during the COVID-19 pandemic [2, 5, 7, 40, 44]. This is worst in doctors who work in the frontline or are of the female gender. This fear in female doctors is also attributed to the fear of infecting members of their families as they are always concerned about their relatives [5, 39].

10. Lack of communication within the health sector: There has been a lack of communication within health systems during the COVID-19 pandemic [2].

Healthcare workers must protect themselves and observe infection, prevention, and control measures to protect themselves from being a source of infection to their family and friends [32]. Employers and managers and management of hospitals need to provide strategies and support doctors, especially those working in the frontline during the COVID-19 pandemic [24, 32].

1.7 Literature review

Several studies have been conducted on the impact of the COVID-19 pandemic on the mental physical and psychological well-being of doctors. These studies have revealed that as long as the COVID-19 pandemic exists, the healthcare provider will continue to experience mental health illnesses including survivors of the SARS-Cov-2 infection [42].

A study conducted in South India among doctors showed that there was a higher prevalence of anxiety and depression among physicians who attended to patients infected with SARS-CoV-2 and were working on the frontline [42]. It was high among primary healthcare doctors compared with doctors working in medical colleges or private hospitals. This may be since doctors working in medical colleges and private hospitals do not have much contact with patients suspected or confirmed with SARS-CoV-2. In this study, doctors work in the primary health center. Since the COVID-19 pandemic does not have enough hours to sleep, they are now working long hours with a heavy workload. In this study, low anxiety was experienced by 86% of the doctors while low and moderate anxiety was experienced by 40% of the respondents [42].

In a study conducted by Lai et al., in China, in 2020, psychological distress occurs in healthcare professionals who have been exposed to COVID-19 including doctors [40]. In this study, the mental health symptoms experienced by the respondents are depression 50.4%, anxiety 44.6%, insomnia 34.0%, and psychological distress 71.5% [40].

A study conducted among junior doctors working at a tertiary London hospital revealed that 34% had concerns relating to their health while 71% and disruptions in their sleep patterns and lifestyle [24].

A systematic review conducted on the impact of the COVID-19 pandemic on the wellness of health professionals revealed that burnout, stress, and emotional burden arise from the task healthcare workers are assigned to taking care of ill patients occurred even before the COVID-19 pandemic [32]. Therefore, doctors and other categories of healthcare workers need to take work-life and work-family life seriously and personally to achieve good mental health.

A study carried out in central, eastern, and western regions of Saudi Arabia, among different categories of healthcare workers and also those working in the ministry of health-owned centers, revealed that 26–19% of the respondents experienced normal depression while 50–83% experienced normal depression [39]. The mental health symptoms experienced by the healthcare workers are anxiety, depression, and insomnia. These symptoms were worst among the female healthcare workers compared with their male counterparts. However, males suffered more psychological distress than female healthcare workers. Therefore, the mental health of healthcare workers at the workplace needs to be addressed. This can be achieved by healthcare workers themselves and also their employers and managers of healthcare [39].

The British Medical Association (BMA) conducted a survey on the well-being of healthcare workers'. The result of this survey revealed that one in five doctors revealed that access to the help that is required is lacking [31]. The British Medical Association also conducted a national study in 2018. This 2018 study showed that about 80% of physicians, mainly junior and middle-grade doctors, experienced burnout, which manifests as exhaustion, depersonalization, and reduced personal efficiency [34]. High-stress levels were experienced by junior and middle-grade doctors working in a district general hospital in Southeast England while investigating the relationship between the COVID-19 pandemic and work-life balance and physical and mental burnout. Three-quarters of the respondents in this survey experienced stress, but hardly accessed support at the workplace [34]. In another survey conducted by the BMA, on the effect of COVID-19 pandemic had on the well-being of doctors [45]. COVID-19 has caused a lot of anxiety, emotional exhaustion, and distress among doctors. Some of the factors that led to this change in work schedule are fear of contracting the SARS-CoV-2 as a nosocomial infection, concerns about personal protective equipment and anxiety over contracting the SARS-CoV-2 and passing it to family members, high mortality of COVID-19 patients, and watching patient caregivers grieve over the loss of their loved ones. Results of this BMA study revealed that 41% of doctors experienced anxiety, burnout, depression, stress, emotional distress, and other symptoms of mental health disorders, which have been worsened by the work of medical practitioners. In this survey, the symptoms of mental health disorders became worst by the COVID-19 in 29% of the doctors surveyed [45].

In an Ireland study, there was a decline in the mental well-being of doctors who experienced anxiety, emotional exhaustion, guilt, isolation, and less support. The respondents had poor well-being [43].

In the United States, there was 49% abnormality in the perceived stress score PSS-4 score in a study on the effect COVID-19 had on the mental health of healthcare workers [6]. In this study, more female respondents (69%) experienced more stress compared with their male counterparts. Depression was experienced by 49% of the healthcare workers surveyed [6].

In Wuhan, China, 522 healthcare workers were surveyed in Fangcang shelter hospitals in 2020, on the effect of the COVID-19 pandemic. Posttraumatic stress disorder, anxiety, depression, insomnia, and distress were experienced by a high rate of the respondents [12]. In this study symptoms of mental health disorder experienced were 25.3% posttraumatic stress disorder, 51.0% anxiety, 58.0% depression, 14.8% insomnia, and 39.1% distress [12].

In a survey conducted in Toronto, Canada, at two different sites of Sinai Health Centre in 2020, there was an increased burnout and psychological distress experienced by the healthcare workers [15]. Among nurses, 54.3% experienced severe emotional exhaustion, and among other healthcare workers severe exhaustion. Results of the study necessitate the need that the provocative and protective factors should be identified [15].

Khoodoruth et al. studied the effect of the COVID-19 pandemic on the mental health of medical residents [9]. In this study, mental health symptoms were experienced by 42.5% depression, 41.7% anxiety, and 30.7% stress. The impact of the COVID-19 pandemic on the mental health of junior residents was worst affected by the negative impact of the COVID-19 pandemic on mental health [9]. Healthcare administrators and managers need to provide support for their employees.

An Australian and New Zealand study investigated the well-being of critical care health professionals during the COVID-19 pandemic [1]. Three themes were identified to improve the well-being of the healthcare professionals, which include providing enough resources to achieve their job role, continuous provision of uncomplicated and comprehensive instructions, and provision of well-being and mental health support services [1].

Physicians' experience during the COVID-19 pandemic was studied, in Lahore, Pakistan. The physical and psychological stress associated with caring for patients infected with SARS-CoV-2 was identified as a challenge the physicians experienced, physicians working in hospitals dedicated to the management of COVID-19 patients were studied [2]. In another study also conducted in Lahore, Pakistan, on the challenges female healthcare workers encounter during the COVID-19 pandemic, some of the challenges experienced by the female healthcare workers were anxiety in caring for patients infected with SAR-CoV-2, empathy toward COVID-19 patients [8]. Female healthcare workers who were not quarantined or isolated after they had contact with COVID-19 patients were more afraid of contracting the novel virus and transmitting it to their households. This is because of the roles assigned to women by their families; therefore, there is a conflict between their family and work life [8].

Junior doctors working in St. George's Hospital London, which is a tertiary health facility in London, were studied in 2020 to access the impact of the COVID-19 pandemic on the training and well-being of the doctors [24]. In this study being healthy was a cause of concern for 34% of the junior doctors studied. There was a change in the sleep pattern of 70% of the juniors and became the worst as the pandemic progressed on 67% of the doctors. The junior doctors were more anxious about transmitting the infection to their household than contracting the SARS-CoV-2 itself [24].

In Oman, a study that investigated the mental health of healthcare professionals revealed that severe anxiety was experienced by the younger ones and women compared with the men and older healthcare workers [16]. The healthcare workers in Oman experienced high-stress levels during the COVID-19 pandemic, which were higher in women, younger healthcare professionals, and healthcare workers working directly involved in the treatment of patients infected with SARS-CoV-2. This is expected as anyone who comes directly in contact with a person infected with the novel virus is at risk of contracting it although the risk is reduced if the healthcare workers use the appropriate personal protective equipment correctly [16].

In Bangladesh, during the COVID-19 pandemic, healthcare workers encountered anxiety, depression, insomnia, and fear of contracting the novel virus and losing their lives to it [35]. Worsened mental stress on the healthcare workers was them infecting members of their families than them contracting it. A contributor to insomnia experienced by some of the healthcare workers in Bangladesh was watching other healthcare workers who contracted the novel virus die. The psychological pressure was caused by ingratitude by other health care workers. The healthcare workers prioritize their patients' health to their well-being. Therefore, the healthcare workers as much as possible practiced infection prevention and control to prevent them from contracting the COVID-19 infection in the medical workplace. In addition, families and friends provided support to improve their mental health [35]. The mental and physical health of healthcare workers must be preserved during the COVID-19 pandemic.

Saeed et al. investigated anxiety and stress among physicians working in the Erbil, Iraqi, Kurdistan region of Iraq in 2020 during the COVID-19 pandemic. In this study the stress level was perceived as 15.4% law stress, 67.3% moderate stress, and 17.3% high stress; there was a significant relationship between the female gender and moderate stress. Physician in this Iraqi study did not experience any form of anxiety was 9.5% while 28.4% severe anxiety [13]. General practitioners and physicians working in health facilities dedicated to the treatment of COVID-19 patients exhibited a higher level of moderate and severe anxiety. Strategies must be taken to decrease the risk at which physicians experience anxiety and stress during the COVID-19 pandemic [13].

In the United Arab Emirates, a study was conducted in three health facilities among healthcare workers at the peak of the COVID-19 pandemic to access their level of anxiety and psychological distress [4]. In this study moderate/severe psychological distress was experienced by 37% of the healthcare workers. Moderate and severe anxiety was experienced by 32.3% of the healthcare workers with 36% of the healthcare workers working on the frontline experiencing a higher anxiety level. The prediction of anxiety and psychological distress was not affected by the wealth of knowledge of COVID-19 the healthcare worker had. The mental health symptom was worst in healthcare workers who had disbelief about the treatment of COVID-19. There was a positive relationship between symptoms and the fear of infecting family members and stigmatization. Psychological distress was exhibited more by healthcare workers who desired psychological support at the workplace. Two-thirds of the healthcare workers in this study experienced anxiety and about 50% had psychological distress and significant numbers both had anxiety and psychological distress. Women healthcare workers in this study were more worried about contracting the novel virus than the men. The factors that affected anxiety and psychological distress in this study are the female genders, transmitting the novel virus to members of their household, stigmatization, and isolation [4].

A systematic review was conducted to investigate the well-being of general practitioners during the COVID-19 pandemic and identified some sources of stress that are affecting physicians [44]. The stressors include altered work schedule, exposure to the SARS-CoV-2, therefore, leading to the increased risk of contracting it, information about COVID-19, lack of organizational and national preparedness, communication gap, lack and shortage of medical supplies and personal protective equipment (PPE), lack of mental support [44]. The mental health problems experienced during the COVID-19 pandemic are stress, anxiety, burnout, fear, depression, and post anxiety, burnout, fear, depression, and posttraumatic stress disorder [44]. The pandemic has also caused job dissatisfaction among physicians. Female doctors have experienced a higher level of mental health symptoms than male doctors. In this review, anxiety and depression were noticed in the younger doctors while stress was experienced more in the older doctor. This increased perceived stress in older healthcare workers was linked to the addition of assigning roles to them, which may include managerial tasks [44].

Steps needed to be taken to reduce mental health symptoms among doctors. The medical workplace should be safe at all times for physicians to work efficiently. The well-being of the populace and especially healthcare workers is threatened by an outbreak of an infectious disease [13]. Poor well-being of healthcare workers including doctors leads to emotional exhaustion. This in turn gives rise to medical errors and litigation, lack of compassion toward patients, low productivity, and increased rate of turnover and work-life imbalance. Patients may also be dissatisfied as they face the reality of the COVID-19 pandemic [33]. Before the COVID-19 pandemic, doctors experienced job stress and this was predicted by job dissatisfaction and poor mental health. The physical and mental well-being of doctors including their mental health of doctors needs improvement by the provision of essential resources and supplies in regard to food at the workplace, which should be without or reduced charge, training on the use of personal protective equipment, child care services, a means of transportation to the hospital during restriction of movement due to the COVID-19 [29], and clear and regular communications. The physicians can be provided with mental and psychological support through telephone calls, telepsychiatry, and provision of mental health insurance and relief for those working in the frontline in the frontline, especially in isolation centers and hospitals dedicated to the treatment of patients with COVID-19 [29].

2. Conclusions

Several changes have been caused by the COVID-19 pandemic. It has affected the mental and physical well-being of doctors negatively. Doctors have developed poor well-being, which has also affected their work. The work of the medical practitioner is a stressful one, which has been made worst by the COVID-19 pandemic. Some of the effects of the pandemic on the mental well-being of doctors are anxiety, burnout depression, distress, and posttraumatic stress disorder. Hospital administrators and managers need to regularly provide mental health support services to physicians as long as the COVID-19 pandemic lasts. Female physicians and physicians working in the frontline are the worst affected.

Conflict of interest

There is no conflict of interest to declare.

Author details

Dabota Yvonne Buowari
Department of Accident and Emergency, University of Port Harcourt Teaching Hospital, Port Harcourt, Nigeria

*Address all correspondence to: dabotabuowari@yahoo.com

References

[1] Elliot R, Crowe L, Bach SW, Abbenbroek B, Grattan S, Hammond NE. Critical care health professionals self-reported needs for well-being during the COVID-19 pandemic: A thematic analysis of the survey. Australian Critical Care. 2022;**35**:40-45

[2] Haq W, Said F, Batool S, Awais HM. Experience of physicians during COVID-19 in a developing country: A qualitative study of Pakistan. The Journal of Infection in Developing Countries. 2021;**15**(2):191-197

[3] World Health Organization. Coronavirus Disease (COVID-19) Outbreak: Rights, Roles and Responsibilities of Health Workers Including Key Considerations for Occupational Safety and Health. Available from: http://www.who.int

[4] Saddik B, Elbarazi L, Temsah MH, Sahib SF, Kheder W, Hussein NA, et al. Psychological distress and anxiety levels among healthcare workers at the height of the COVID-19 pandemic in the United Arab Emirates. International Journal of Public Health. 2020;**66**:1604367. DOI: 10.3389/ijph.2021.1604369

[5] Kock JH, Latham HA, Leslies J, Grindle M, Munoz S, Ellis L, et al. A rapid review of the impact of COVID-19 on the mental health of healthcare workers: Implications for supporting psychological wellbeing. BMC Public Health. 2021;**21**:104. DOI: 10.1186/s12889-020-10070-3

[6] Aiyer A, Surani S, Ratnani I, Surani S. Mental health impact of COVID-19 on healthcare workers in the USA: A cross-sectional web-based survey. Journal of Depression and Anxiety. 2020;**9**(373):1-8. DOI: 10.35248/2162-1044.20.9.373

[7] Muller AE, Hafstad EV, Himmels JPW, Smedslund G, Flottorp S, Stensland S, et al. The mental health impact of the COVID-19 pandemic on healthcare workers and interventions to help them: A rapid systematic review. Psychiatry Research. 2020;**293**:113441. DOI: 10.1016/j.psychres.2020.113441

[8] Shahbaz S, Ashraf MZ, Zakar R, Fischer F. Psychological, emotional and professional challenges faced by female healthcare professionals during the COVID-19 outbreak in Lahore, Pakistan: A qualitative study. BMC Women's Health. 2020;**21**:197. DOI: 10.1186/s12905-021-01344.y

[9] Khoodoruth MAS, Al-Nuaimi SK, Al-Salihy Z, Ghaffar A, Khoodoruth WNC, Ouanes S. Factors associated with mental health outcomes among medical residents exposed to COVID-19. BJPsych. 2021;**7**(e52):1-6. DOI: 10.1192/bjo.2021.12

[10] Madhuchandra MK, Srimathi NL. Psychological well-being among doctors and nurses: A comparative study. The International Journal of Indian Psychology. 2016;**3**(4):68

[11] Adealu JO, Yussuf OB, Popoola OA. Prevalence and correlates of job stress among junior doctors in the university college hospital, Ibadan. Annals of Ibadan Postgraduate Medicine. 2016;**14**:92-98

[12] Gui Y, Zhu Y, Xu G. Factors associated with mental health outcomes among healthcare workers in the Fangcang shelter Hospital in China. International Journal of Social Psychiatry. 2020;**68**(1):1-9

[13] Saeed AE, Shabila NP, Aziz AJ. Stress and anxiety among physicians during

the COVID-19 outbreak in the Iraqi Kurdistan region: An online survey. PLoS One. 2021;**16**(6):e0253903. DOI: 10.1371/journal.prone.02533903

[14] Villain L, Pastorina R, Molinari E, Anelli F, Ricciardi IV, Graffigna G, et al. Impact of the COVID-19 pandemic on the psychological wellbeing of students in an Italian university: A web-based cross-sectional survey. Globalization and Health. 2021;**17**:39. DOI: 10.1186/s12992-021-00680-w

[15] Maunder RG, Heeney ND, Kiss A, Hunter JJ, Jeffs LP, Ginty L, et al. Psychological impact of the COVID-19 pandemic on hospital workers overtime: Relationship to occupational role living with children and elders, and modifiable factors. General Hospital Psychiatry. 2021;**71**:88-94

[16] Badahdah A, Khamis F, Mahyijari NA, Balushi MA, Hatmi HA, Salmi A, et al. The mental health of health care workers in Oman during the COVID-19 pandemic. International Journal of Social Psychiatry. 2021;**67**(1):90-95

[17] Ohia C, Bakarey AS, Ahmad T. COVID-19 and Nigeria: Putting the realities in context. International Journal of Infectious Diseases. 2020;**95**:279-281

[18] Rehman MF, Fariba C, Anwar A, Shalizad N, Ahmad M, Mukhtar S, et al. Novel coronavirus disease (COVID-19) pandemic: A recent mini-review. Computational and Structural Biotechnological Journal. 2021;**19**:612-623

[19] World Health Organization. Mental Health and Psychological Considerations during the COVID-19 Outbreak. www.who.int [Accessed: March 18, 2020]

[20] Sesio S, Buomprisco G, La Torre G, et al. The impact of COVID-19 on doctors' wellbeing: Results of a web survey during the lockdown in Italy. Europe Review Medicine Pharmacology Science. 2020;**24**:7869-7879. Available from: http://www.europeanreview.org

[21] Cairns P, Aitken G, Popel M, Cecil JE, Cunningham KB, Ferguson J, et al. Interventions for the wellbeing of healthcare workers during a pandemic or other crisis: Scoping review. BMJ Open. 2021;**11**:e047498. DOI: 10.1136/bmjopen-2020-047498

[22] Khan M, Adil SF, Alkhathlan HZ, Tahir MN, Saif S, Khan M, et al. COVID-19: A global challenge with old history, epidemiology and progress so far. Molecules. 2021;**26**:39. DOI: 10.3390/molecules26010039

[23] Simons Q, Baldwin DS. A critical review of the definition of 'wellbeing for doctors and their patients in a post-COVID-19 era. International Journal of Social Psychiatry. 2021;**67**(8):984-991

[24] Salem J, Hawkins L, Gates J, Sundaran A, Ong YE, Fernando A, et al. COVID-19 and the impact on doctor well-being and training - a mixed-methods study. The Physician. 2020;**6**(3):108. Epub05.10.2020. DOI: 1038192/1.6.3.2

[25] Sfeatcu R, Cermusca-Mitariu M, LonescuC, RomanM, Cermusca-MitariuS, Coldea L, et al. The concept of wellbeing in relation to health and quality of life. European Journal of Science and Theology. 2014;**10**(4):123-128

[26] World Medical Association. The Physicians Pledge. Available from: https://www.wma.net/policies.post/wma.declaration-of-geneva

[27] Kim R. World Health Organization and Wellbeing at Work. Available from: http://www.who.int

[28] Brooks SK, Gerada C, Chalder T. Review of literature on the mental health of doctors: Are specialist services needed. Journal of Mental Health. 2011;**20**(2):1-11

[29] Pandemic Workforce Well-Being. A Comprehensive Toolkit for Supporting our Own During COVID-19. Mount Sinai. Available from: http://www.owbr@mssm.edu

[30] Galbraith N, Boyda D, McFeeters D, Hassan T. The mental health of doctors during the COVID-19 pandemic. BJPsych Bulletin. 2020;**45**(2):93-97. DOI: 10.1192/bjb.2020.44

[31] World Health Organization. The Impact of COVID-19 on Health and Care Workers a Closer Look at Deaths. Health Workforce Department Working Paper 1. Geneva: World Health Organization; 2021 (WHO/HWF/workingpaper/20201). Licence: CCBY-NC-SA-3.0190

[32] Shreffler J, Petrey J, Huecker M. The impact of COVID-19 on healthcare worker wellness: A scoping review. Western Journal of Emergency Medicine. 2020;**21**(5):1059-1066

[33] Johnson J, Simms-Ellis R, Janes G, Mills T, Budworth L, Atkinson L, et al. Can we prepare healthcare professionals and students for involvement in stressful healthcare events? A mixed-methods evaluation of a resilience training intervention. BMC Health Services Research. 2020;**20**:1094. DOI: 10.1186/s12913-020-05948-2

[34] Revythis A, Shoh S, Enyioma C, Ghose A, Patel M, Karathana A, et al. The experience of a single NHS England trust on the trust on the impact of the COVID-19 pandemic on junior and middle-grade doctors. What is next? International Journal of Environmental Research and Public Health. 2021;**18**:1041. DOI: 10.3390/ijerph/181910413

[35] Razu SR, Yasmin T, Arif TB, Islam S, Islam SMS, Gesesew HA, et al. Challenges faced by healthcare professionals during the COVID-19 pandemic: A qualitative inquiry from Bangladesh. Frontiers in Public Health. 2021;**9**:1-8. DOI: 10.3389/fpubh.2021.1647315

[36] British Medical Association. The Mental Health and Wellbeing of the Medical Workforce - Now and Beyond COVID-19. Available from: http://www.bma.org.uk/covid19

[37] Goddard AF, Patel M. The changing face of medical professionalism and the impact of COVID-19. The Lancet. 2021;**397**:397950-397952. Available from: http://www.thelancet.com. DOI: 10.101b/s0140-6736(21)00436-0

[38] Yates SW. Physician stress and burnout. The American Journal of Medicine. 2019;**133**(2):160-164

[39] Ammari AM, Sultana K, Thomas A, Swaidan CA, Harthi NA. Mental health outcomes amongst healthcare workers during the COVID-19 pandemic in Saudi Arabia. Frontiers in Psychiatry. 2021;**11**:1-11. DOI: 10.3389/fpsyt.2020.619540

[40] Lai J, Ma S, Wang Y, Lai Z, Hu Z, Wei N, et al. Factors associated with mental health outcomes among healthcare workers exposed to coronavirus-2019. JAMA Network Open. 2020;**3**(3):e203976. DOI: 10.1001/jamanetworkopen.2020.3976

[41] Schneider J, Talamonti D, Gibson B, Forshaw M. Factors mediating the psychological wellbeing of healthcare workers responding to global pandemics. A systematic review. Journal of Health Psychology. 2021:1-22

[42] Veeraragharan V, Srinivasan K. Workplace impact on the mental

wellbeing of the frontline doctor. Journal of Mind and Medical Sciences. 2020;**7**:2. DOI: 10.2254317674.72.P 188192

[43] Creese J, Byrne P, Conway E, Barett E, Prithodova L, Humphries N. 'We all really need to just take a breath'. Composite narratives of hospital doctors' wellbeing during the COVID-19 pandemic. International Journal of Environmental Research and Public Health. 2021;**18**:2051. DOI: 10.3390/ijerph/18042051

[44] Jefferson L, Golder S, Heathcote C, Avila AC, Date V, Essex H, et al. General physicians wellbeing during the COVID-19 pandemic: A systematic review. British Journal of General Practice. 2022;**72**(718):e325-e333. DOI: 10.3399/BJGP.2021.0680

[45] Hospital Times. BMA Survey Reveals the Effects of Covid-19 on Doctors' Well-being. Available from: http://www.bma.org